Wireless Networks

Series Editor

Xuemin Sherman Shen, University of Waterloo, Waterloo, ON, Canada

The purpose of Springer's Wireless Networks book series is to establish the state of the art and set the course for future research and development in wireless communication networks. The scope of this series includes not only all aspects of wireless networks (including cellular networks, WiFi, sensor networks, and vehicular networks), but related areas such as cloud computing and big data. The series serves as a central source of references for wireless networks research and development. It aims to publish thorough and cohesive overviews on specific topics in wireless networks, as well as works that are larger in scope than survey articles and that contain more detailed background information. The series also provides coverage of advanced and timely topics worthy of monographs, contributed volumes, textbooks and handbooks.

Xiaonan Guo • Yan Wang • Jerry Cheng •
Yingying (Jennifer) Chen

Mobile Technologies for Smart Healthcare System Design

Springer

Xiaonan Guo
Department of Information Science and Technology
George Mason University
Fairfax, VA, USA

Yan Wang
Department of Computer and Information Sciences
Temple University
Philadelphia, PA, USA

Jerry Cheng
Department of Computer Science
New York Institute of Technology
New York, NY, USA

Yingying (Jennifer) Chen
Department of Electrical and Computer Engineering
Rutgers University
Piscataway, NJ, USA

ISSN 2366-1186 ISSN 2366-1445 (electronic)
Wireless Networks
ISBN 978-3-031-57347-7 ISBN 978-3-031-57345-3 (eBook)
https://doi.org/10.1007/978-3-031-57345-3

This Springer imprint is published by the registered company Springer Nature Switzerland AG
The registered company address is: Gewerbestrasse 11, 6330 Cham, Switzerland

Preface

Nowadays, people pay more attention to their physical health because the accelerated pace of life and increasing work pressure have compelled many people to adapt to a sedentary lifestyle. Such sedentary lifestyles often lead to many chronic illnesses (e.g., obesity), which negatively impact people's quality of life. Thus, it is important to continuously pay attention to people's health conditions and provide in-time actions. The traditional way of healthcare requires patients to perform hospital visits or wear dedicated devices, which are intrusive and costly. Consequently, solutions providing a low-cost, long-term, non-invasive health monitoring system are highly desirable. Mobile technologies have recently demonstrated success in many application domains, including pervasive computing, Internet of Things (IoT), smart homes, etc. The integrated sensor modalities and wireless communication capabilities make mobile technologies a promising way to address healthcare needs that traditional approaches cannot offer. This book intends to provide comprehensive analyses and state-of-the-art designs of low-cost, long-term, and non-invasive health monitoring systems from different perspectives by leveraging mobile sensing technologies.

In this book, we show how to utilize wireless signals and mobile technologies to facilitate smart healthcare in addition to their original capabilities. In particular, we introduce the identification of many kinds of activities exploiting the prevalence of WiFi infrastructure. We extract channel state information (CSI) in WiFi signals to achieve fine-grained activity recognition. Furthermore, a personalized fitness assistant system in home/office environments has been designed using the existing WiFi infrastructure. Since millimeter wave (mmWave) technologies have already been integrated into WiFi standards, they become a promising solution to enhance the resolution and accuracy of wireless-based smart healthcare systems. Along this direction, the personalized fitness assistant system has been further enhanced by using a single commercial-off-the-shelf (COTS) mmWave device to demonstrate its capability to handle more complex scenarios in indoor environments, including dynamic environment changes and multiple people. We then study another essential healthcare component, eating habit monitoring, which can facilitate dietary behavior analysis and nutrition study. The designed system provides environment-invariant eating behavior monitoring. Moreover, we find that mobile devices (e.g., smartphones and smartwatches) can be extended for smart healthcare in addition to their original usage. We again develop a personalized fitness assistant system for people carrying mobile devices to help them achieve fitness goals while minimizing the chances of injury. The system dynamically depicts comprehensive short-term and long-term workout pictures of the user's exercises using wearable mobile devices. In addition to its original usage of measuring physiological signals, photoplethysmography (PPG) sensors are exploited to facilitate advanced healthcare applications. Specifically, we demonstrate that built-in PPG sensors on wearables can enable finger-level gesture recognition, sign language interpretation, and continuous user authentication.

Fairfax, VA, USA — Xiaonan Guo
Philadelphia, PA, USA — Yan Wang
New York, NY, USA — Jerry Cheng
Piscataway, NJ, USA — Yingying (Jennifer) Chen
November 2023

Contents

Chapter 1
Introduction

1.1 Background

The advent of mobile sensing technologies has facilitated widespread connectivity among different devices, including smartphones, tablets, voice assistants, wireless sensors, and smart appliances. This integration has transformed many aspects of daily life and enabled a wide range of applications such as mobile healthcare monitoring, activity recognition, and user authentication.

In particular, long-term healthcare-related applications employing mobile sensing technologies are crucial in promoting personal well-being. Notably, the portability of mobile devices, coupled with their wearability around the clock, offers continuous monitoring capabilities. These applications are crucial for vulnerable demographics of young children and people suffering from chronic diseases such as obesity, paralysis, or respiratory illnesses. Therefore, sensing methodologies for long-term mobile health monitoring have become essential in diverse research spanning areas such as activity recognition, fitness assistance, dietary tracking, and vital signs monitoring.

To support these functions, various forms of techniques in mobile devices have been developed, each with unique usage potential. Traditionally, health monitoring was primarily conducted in hospitals. These institutions utilized specialized sensors like electrocardiograms or glucometers to track specific aspects of an individual's health, in order to provide comprehensive evaluations. In comparison, choices for home-based monitoring used to be quite limited. Nowadays, users can utilize personal devices such as smartphones or wearable devices to enable the wide adoption of long-term mobile health monitoring in their daily lives. This evolution has been enabled through the integration of diverse sensors. The proliferation of WiFi has interconnected numerous mobile devices, thereby conferring upon each device the ability to offer mobile sensing capabilities. Furthermore, inherent sensors like accelerometers and microphones within mobile devices can augment the sensing capabilities even further.

X. Guo et al., *Mobile Technologies for Smart Healthcare System Design*,
Wireless Networks, https://doi.org/10.1007/978-3-031-57345-3_1

1.1.1 Advanced Mobile Sensing Technologies

1.1.1.1 WiFi-based Technologies

Fine-grained Channel State Information (CSI) has been proposed as a more accurate wireless sensing strategy utilizing WiFi signals. Unlike Received Signal Strength (RSS), CSI not only indicates path loss over distance but also aggregates multipath effects such as scattering and fading. This makes CSI more sensitive to changes in signal propagation caused by human body movement, including subconscious motions associated with breathing [18, 24, 25, 30, 41, 42]. In comparison to RSS, CSI contains a larger set of values, including amplitude and phase information, for orthogonal frequency division multiplexing (OFDM) subcarriers. Separate subcarriers can span different frequency ranges and, thus, experience slightly different multipathing effects while propagating from the WiFi endpoint devices. This information provides more fine-grained details of the wireless channel than RSS. Consequently, CSI has enabled WiFi signals to become a promising sensing modality for healthcare applications.

1.1.1.2 mmWave-based technologies

As mmWave technologies are integrated into WiFi standards, they also emerge as a promising solution to enhance the resolution accuracy in wireless-based smart healthcare systems. mmWave signals have higher frequencies than traditional WiFi signals (i.e., 2.4 and 5 GHz). They typically operate in the tens to hundreds of GHz range and thus can utilize a broader bandwidth [45]. Although mmWave signals have limitations in penetrating materials and long-range transmissions due to shorter wavelengths, their sensitivity to environmental changes can be highly advantageous in fine-grained sensing. Such features allow mmWave signals to detect subtle movements caused by heartbeat and breathing, making them an excellent choice for advanced smart health applications. Futhermore, the smaller antenna array used in mmWave transmission allows these systems to remain portable and easy to integrate into mobile healthcare sensing systems.

1.1.1.3 Inertial Sensor-based Technologies

Motion sensors, including accelerometers, gyroscopes, and magnetometers, can detect linear accelerations, rotational rate, and force along 2–6 degrees of freedom, depending on levels of sophistication. Furthermore, motion sensors find frequent utilization in commercial items like smartphones and wearable devices. These sensors are often integrated into Inertial Measurement Units (IMUs) to adhere to compact size prerequisites. To maintain high accuracy, accelerometers, gyroscopes, and magnetometers can be utilized jointly, with each performing a different function. Accelerometers function by generating electrical charges, which are proportional to the force of vibration or contraction, based on the piezoelectric effect [19]. Since the mass of the device remains constant, the generated charge is proportional to the acceleration and can be utilized to derive linear indications of position, such as velocity or distance. Gyroscopes, on the other hand, provide additional information on the axis of rotation by measuring low-current electrical signals produced by an internal rotor [35]. These sensors are susceptible to accumulating errors over time, which can result in a drifting effect when further calculations are made using flawed measurements.

Data from motion sensors is one of the most straightforward and comprehensible metrics, and as a result, many basic mobile health monitoring systems utilize this data to provide a quantifiable trace of an individual's physical activity [32, 34]. Studies have demonstrated that patterns in motion data can indicate periodic motions and gestures associated with walking, running, stretching, breathing, and other activities [10]. This data can be gathered using standalone sensors or by utilizing existing devices such as smartphones, smartwatches, and fitness trackers [14, 26].

1.1.1.4 PPG-based Technologies

Photoplethysmography (PPG) is an optical technique that measures blood volume changes through light reflection or absorption from the skin and underlying tissues. A typical PPG setup involves shining single-frequency light from an LED onto the skin and measuring the absorbed or reflected light with a photodiode [33]. Traditionally, PPG data is instrumental in determining heart rates, pulse oximetry, and heart rhythm irregularities. In existing health monitoring systems, PPG measurements are known to be susceptible to body motion artifacts, which generate interference in blood volumes and reduce system performance. However, recent studies showed that such motion artifacts can be leveraged to analyze muscle movements, expanding the use of PPG to more smart healthcare-related applications, including sign language interpretation and user authentication.

1.1.2 Mobile Healthcare Systems

1.1.2.1 Daily Activity Recognition

Activity recognition plays a crucial role in long-term mobile healthcare systems, particularly in monitoring Activities of Daily Living (ADLs). It allows for non-intrusive tracking of a patient's routine activities and physical state, providing valuable insights into their health and well-being. Furthermore, the significance of activity recognition extends to being a foundational element upon which other functionalities such as fitness monitoring, eating tracking, and more are constructed. By identifying pre-defined patterns in sensory data, activity recognition can monitor a user's daily tasks, such as eating, dressing, and moving around [4, 20], as well as their postures [2, 31]. It can also detect potential health risks, such as falls [5]. This information not only offers a comprehensive view of the patient's daily functioning and independence but can also aid in early detection and prevention of health issues.

Smartwatches [37], sensor networks [44], and mobile phones [37] are all devices that can be used for device-based activity recognition. These devices can be worn or carried by the patient, allowing for easy tracking of their body motions. Additionally, hardware such as mobile phones and WiFi access points can be repurposed for device-free activity recognition [43, 47], enabling the monitoring of patients at a distance.

Integrating activity recognition into mobile healthcare systems, particularly for monitoring Activities of Daily Living (ADLs), can significantly enhance mobile healthcare. This technology allows healthcare providers to understand a patient's daily routines and physical habits, enabling them to offer personalized care based on the patient's unique lifestyle and needs. By tracking these daily activities, early signs of potential health issues can be detected, allowing for timely intervention before they escalate into serious problems. This proactive approach not only improves patient outcomes but also enhances the quality of life for patients by promoting independence and maintaining their daily functionalities.

1.1.2.2 Fitness Assistance

Different from regular activity recognition, smart fitness assistance systems place emphasis on providing personalized guidance and support to users during their fitness activities. These systems often integrate wearable devices or smartphone applications that collect data related to heart rate, calorie expenditure, distance covered, and other relevant metrics. By processing this information, smart fitness assistance systems can offer real-time feedback, exercise recommendations, and progress tracking to enhance the effectiveness of workouts and improve overall fitness levels.

Sustaining fitness is a vital aspect for individuals engaged in activities such as regular gym visits and the general public. The dynamic nature of exercise calls for portable sensing solutions to accurately monitor and adapt to their active routines. As users may be moving quickly in larger public spaces such as gyms or outdoors, fitness assistance systems tend to prefer small, device-based solutions [28, 48]. However, device-free methods can still function well in indoor scenarios [46, 50]. With the increasing demand for personalized healthcare, smart fitness assistance systems have the potential to become an essential component in the overall mobile healthcare ecosystem.

1.1.2.3 Daily Dietary Tracking

One of the primary concerns for nutritionists is to develop and verify adherence to a daily dietary plan for their clients [17]. With the increasing stress at work and fast-paced lifestyles, people are more prone to forming unhealthy habits, particularly unhealthy eating habits, which can lead to various illnesses. According to a survey by the World Health Organization, more than 1.9 billion adults worldwide are overweight, and 650 million are obese. These people are at risk for dietary health problems [23]. Therefore, finding solutions to diet-related issues is an urgent matter, and efficient daily dietary tracking is a necessity.

Monitoring eating behaviors, such as food types, quantities, and eating speed, can provide valuable insights into an individual's diet and health status. Traditional methods for tracking daily dietary intake require self-reporting from the users [7, 12, 13, 16, 40]. However, self-reporting can be inconvenient and inaccurate due to the user's lack of experience in recording nutritional content or forgetfulness in making timely log updates.

To address these limitations, there have been a recent surge of research on automatic dietary monitoring. Vision-based approaches that use cameras to capture food information, such as photos or videos of meals, have been proposed [38]. Kong et al. [22] suggest using the user's mobile device to take photo strings or short videos to perform automatic dietary assessment. Zhu et al. [49] provide an image analysis method to recognize eating and evaluate food amount and type. O'Liughlin et al. [29] explore the feasibility of using the Microsoft SenseCam [15] to estimate dietary energy intake in various sports populations.

Beyond just relying on vision-based techniques, the prevalence of wearable devices integrated with diverse sensors has surged, serving as effective tools for tracking daily dietary intake. This book will delve into the utilization of mmWave technology for the purpose of monitoring daily dietary intake, as dietary tracking involves capturing gestures on a smaller scale. The application of mmWave technology is well-suited for this task due to its capacity to offer high-resolution insights.

1.1.2.4 Fine-grained Sign Language Recognition

The demand for wrist-worn wearable devices has witnessed a remarkable surge since 2015, with an estimated global shipment of 101.4 million units in 2019 [21]. This increasing popularity of wrist-worn wearables opens up exciting opportunities to harness diverse sensing modalities for pervasive hand or finger gesture recognition. Hand and finger gestures encompass a wide spectrum of combinations, providing rich information that can power numerous intricate human-computer interaction (HCI) applications. These applications include wearable controls, virtual reality (VR)/augmented reality (AR) systems, and automatic sign language translation. To illustrate the potential of automatic sign language translation, consider a wrist-worn wearable device like a smartwatch or a wristband. Equipped with sensors, it can convert sign language into audio and text, and vice versa. This technology holds immense promise in facilitating communication between individuals who are deaf or have hearing difficulties and those who are unfamiliar with sign language. A recent review conducted by Er-Rady et al. [6] sheds light on the existing methods of automatic sign language translation, which are still in their early stages. This review serves as a driving force for us to develop a robust finger-level gesture recognition system that can effectively address this challenge.

1.1.2.5 User Identification and User Authentication

User Identification and User Authentication are crucial components of ensuring secure access to systems and protecting sensitive information. User identification refers to the process of uniquely identifying individual users within a system or application. This is typically achieved through recognizing unique identifiers. User authentication, on the other hand, involves verifying the identity of a user to ensure that they are who they claim to be. This verification process is essential for granting access to resources or restricted areas that are exclusively designated for authorized users. Common authentication methods include passwords, biometric authentication (such as fingerprint or facial recognition), and two-factor authentication. The combination of robust user identification and authentication mechanisms play a vital role in preventing unauthorized access, protecting user privacy, and safeguarding sensitive data from malicious actors.

Recently, there is a growing body of research and development focusing on utilizing mobile devices for user identification and authentication. For instance, gesture recognition is emerging as a promising approach in this field. To establish user identity, gesture recognition algorithms analyze the unique patterns and characteristics of individual gestures [9, 36]. These algorithms can distinguish between authorized users and impostors by assessing factors like gesture speed, duration, direction, and shape. Furthermore, behavioral biometrics, such as keystroke dynamics [1, 3, 8] and gait analysis [11, 27, 39], concentrate on the distinctive behavioral patterns exhibited by individuals. These methods monitor factors such as typing rhythms, touchscreen gestures, or walking patterns to establish and authenticate user identity.

1.2 Challenges

In this section, we will further discuss the challenging issues in designing long-term mobile healthcare systems.

1.2.1 Issues in Raw Data Collection for Mobile Healthcare

Utilizing mobile technologies and mobile sensing for applications like activity recognition, fitness monitoring, eating monitoring, user identification, and user authentications introduce numerous data collection challenges. The complexity and diversity of human activities demand highly accurate and reliable sensors, yet sensor limitations, including signal variability, noise, and drift, often impact data integrity. Moreover, activities such as eating or exercising may result in drastic changes in body motion and physiological signals, which can further complicate data interpretation. When it comes to fitness tracking, the data collected from different individuals can vary significantly due to personal factors such as age, gender, fitness level, and health status, making it challenging to design universally applicable algorithms. For user identification and authentication applications, issues like false positives and negatives, and spoofing attacks are major concerns. Besides, privacy and security are of great importance, given the sensitivity of the data collected, yet ensuring these while providing seamless user experiences can be challenging. In addition, dealing with the large volume of data generated by continuous monitoring, along with battery life considerations for mobile devices, adds another layer of complexity to these applications.

1.2.2 Extracting Effective Features for Designing Mobile Heathcare System

Another challenges of employing mobile technologies for mobile healthcare related applications in feature extraction. Feature extraction is crucial for transforming raw sensor data into meaningful information, but achieving this reliably and accurately is a complex task. For applications like activity recognition and fitness monitoring, the dynamic nature of human activities demands robust features that can capture unique patterns amid a wide range of movements and physiological responses. Selecting the right features is equally challenging, particularly when it comes to recognizing diverse eating behaviors or authenticating users based on biometric data. The variability between individuals' behaviors or biometric patterns requires the extraction of highly discriminative features to ensure accurate identification and authentication. Furthermore, extracted features should be resistant to noise and sensor errors, which is challenging given the inherent variability in mobile environments. Another obstacle is computational efficiency. Mobile devices have limited processing capabilities, so feature extraction methods need to be optimized to function effectively under these constraints. Finally, ensuring privacy while extracting meaningful features from sensitive data is a delicate balance that requires sophisticated strategies and protocols.

1.2.3 Enhancing System Robustness in Practical Environments

When designing long-term mobile healthcare system, environmental changes also pose significant challenges. Mobile devices are often used in diverse and dynamically changing environments, which can significantly affect the quality and accuracy of the system. For example, activity recognition and fitness monitoring may be influenced by changes in lighting, weather, terrain, and user context, such as indoor versus outdoor activities. These changes can introduce variations in sensor data that may not necessarily correspond to changes in the user's activity, leading to misinterpretations. Similarly, for eating monitoring, different environments like restaurants, homes, or offices could impact user behavior, and hence the sensor data. User identification and authentication systems also have to contend with environmental variations, such as changes in ambient noise that could affect voice recognition, or lighting changes impacting facial recognition. Furthermore, environmental factors can also affect the device's performance itself, for instance, temperature fluctuations influencing battery life, or signal strength variation due to changes in location. Therefore, designing robust systems that can adapt and respond to these environmental changes remains a major challenge for mobile sensing applications.

1.3 Book Organization

The book commences with an introduction in Chap. 1 that gives an overview of the content, followed by a detailed discussion on the background of the topic. It specifically covers advanced mobile sensing technologies and mobile healthcare system design. This section sets the context and highlights the importance of the subject matter. Subsequently, the challenges and contributions to the field are presented, with the organization of the book succinctly outlined. The book then delves into detailed chapters on specific topics including contactless activity identification using commercial WiFi in Chap. 2, personalized fitness assistance using commodity WiFi in Chap. 3, multi-person fitness assistance via millimeter wave in Chap. 4, non-intrusive eating habits derivation using millimeter wave in Chap. 4, Fitness Assistance Using Motion Sensor in Chap. 6, Fine-grained gesture recognition and sign language interpretation via PPG on smartwatches in Chap. 7 and continuous user authentication via PPG in Chap. 8. Each of these chapters starts with a background study, related works, and detailed system design with its implementation and evaluation. In conclusion, the book integrates cutting-edge technologies and novel methodologies to provide a comprehensive understanding of mobile sensing technologies and long-term mobile healthcare systems.

References

1. Alsultan, A., Warwick, K., Wei, H.: Non-conventional keystroke dynamics for user authentication. Pattern Recogn. Lett. **89**, 53–59 (2017)
2. Baek, J., Yun, B.J.: Posture monitoring system for context awareness in mobile computing. IEEE Trans. Instrum. Meas. **59**(6), 1589–1599 (2010)

3. Çeker, H., Upadhyaya, S.: User authentication with keystroke dynamics in long-text data. In: 2016 IEEE 8th International Conference on Biometrics Theory, Applications and Systems (BTAS), pp. 1–6. IEEE (2016)
4. Chen, L., Hoey, J., Nugent, C.D., Cook, D.J., Yu, Z.: Sensor-based activity recognition. IEEE Trans. Syst. Man. Cybern. Part C (Appl. Rev.) **42**(6), 790–808 (2012)
5. Damodaran, N., Haruni, E., Kokhkharova, M., Schäfer, J.: Device free human activity and fall recognition using wifi channel state information (csi). CCF Trans. Pervasive Comput. Interact. **2**, 1–17 (2020)
6. Er-Rady, A., Faizi, R., Thami, R.O.H., Housni, H.: Automatic sign language recognition: a survey. In: 2017 International Conference on Advanced Technologies for Signal and Image Processing (ATSIP), pp. 1–7. IEEE (2017)
7. Fallaize, R., Forster, H., Macready, A.L., Walsh, M.C., Mathers, J.C., Brennan, L., Gibney, E.R., Gibney, M.J., Lovegrove, J.A.: Online dietary intake estimation: reproducibility and validity of the food4me food frequency questionnaire against a 4-day weighed food record. J. Med. Internet Res. **16**(8), e190 (2014)
8. Feng, T., Zhao, X., Carbunar, B., Shi, W.: Continuous mobile authentication using virtual key typing biometrics. In: 2013 12th IEEE International Conference on Trust, Security and Privacy in Computing and Communications, pp. 1547–1552. IEEE (2013)
9. Furnell, S., Clarke, N., Karatzouni, S.: Beyond the pin: Enhancing user authentication for mobile devices. Comput. Fraud Secur. **2008**(8), 12–17 (2008)
10. Ghosh, A.M., Halder, D., Hossain, S.K.A.: Remote health monitoring system through iot. In: 2016 5th International Conference on Informatics, Electronics and Vision (ICIEV), pp. 921–926 (2016)
11. Giorgi, G., Martinelli, F., Saracino, A., Sheikhalishahi, M.: Walking through the deep: gait analysis for user authentication through deep learning. In: ICT Systems Security and Privacy Protection: 33rd IFIP TC 11 International Conference, SEC 2018, Held at the 24th IFIP World Computer Congress, WCC 2018, Poznan, Poland, September 18–20, 2018, Proceedings 33, pp. 62–76. Springer (2018)
12. Hankin, J.H., Wilkens, L.R., Kolonel, L.N., Yoshizawa, C.N.: Validation of a quantitative diet history method in hawaii. Am. J. Epidemiol. **133**(6), 616–628 (1991)
13. Harlan, L.C., Block, G.: Use of adjustment factors with a brief food frequency questionnaire to obtain nutrient values. Epidemiology **1**(3), 224–231 (1990)
14. Hassana, M.M., Uddin, Z., Mohamed, A., Almogrena, A.: A robust human activity recognition system using smartphone sensors and deep learning. Future Gener. Comput. Syst. **81**, 307–313 (2018)
15. Hodges, S., Williams, L., Berry, E., Izadi, S., Srinivasan, J., Butler, A., Smyth, G., Kapur, N., Wood, K.: Sensecam: A retrospective memory aid. In: Dourish, P., Friday, A. (eds.) UbiComp 2006: Ubiquitous Computing, pp. 177–193. Springer Berlin Heidelberg, Berlin, Heidelberg (2006)
16. Jain, M., Howe, G.R., Rohan, T.: Dietary assessment in epidemiology: comparison of a food frequency and a diet history questionnaire with a 7-day food record. Am. J. Epidemiol. **143**(9), 953–960 (1996)
17. Johnson, R.K.: Dietary intake–how do we measure what people are really eating? Obesity **10**(s11), 63S (2002)
18. Khamis, A., Chou, C.T., Kusy, B., Hu, W.: Cardiofi: enabling heart rate monitoring on unmodified cots wifi devices. In: Proceedings of the 15th EAI International Conference on Mobile and Ubiquitous Systems: Computing, Networking and Services, MobiQuitous '18, pp. 97–106. Association for Computing Machinery, New York (2018). https://doi.org/10.1145/3286978.3287003
19. Kim, J.D., Kim, D.S.: Development of a combined-type tool dynamometer with a piezo-film accelerometer for an ultra-precision lathe. J. Mater. Process. Technol. **71**(3), 360–366 (1997)
20. Kim, E., Helal, S., Cook, D.: Human activity recognition and pattern discovery. IEEE Pervasive Comput. **9**(1), 48–53 (2009)

21. Klostermann Klostermann, J.: Blinging up fashionable wearable technologies (2015). https://cloudtweaks.com/2015/11/blinging-up-fashionable-wearable-technologies/
22. Kong, F., Tan, J.: Dietcam: Automatic dietary assessment with mobile camera phones. Pervasive Mob. Comput. **8**(1), 147–163 (2012). https://doi.org/10.1016/j.pmcj.2011.07.003. http://www.sciencedirect.com/science/article/pii/S1574119211001131
23. Lin, Z., Xie, Y., Guo, X., Wang, C., Ren, Y., Chen, Y.: Wi-fi-enabled automatic eating moment monitoring using smartphones. In: International Conference on Internet of Things Technologies for HealthCare 2019 (2020)
24. Liu, J., Wang, Y., Chen, Y., Yang, J., Chen, X., Cheng, J.: Tracking vital signs during sleep leveraging off-the-shelf wifi. In: Proceedings of the 16th ACM International Symposium on Mobile Ad Hoc Networking and Computing, pp. 267–276. ACM (2015)
25. Mahmood Khan, U., Kabir, Z., Hassan, S.A.: Wireless health monitoring using passive wifi sensing. In: 2017 13th International Wireless Communications and Mobile Computing Conference (IWCMC), pp. 1771–1776 (2017)
26. McNamara, L., Ngai, E.: Sadhealth: a personal mobile sensing system for seasonal health monitoring. IEEE Syst. J. **12**(1), 30–40 (2018)
27. Mufandaidza, M., Ramotsoela, T., Hancke, G.P.: Continuous user authentication in smartphones using gait analysis. In: IECON 2018-44th Annual Conference of the IEEE Industrial electronics society, pp. 4656–4661. IEEE (2018)
28. Muneer, A., Fati, S.M., Fuddah, S.: Smart health monitoring system using iot based smart fitness mirror. TELKOMNIKA (Telecommun. Comput. Electron. Control) **18**(1), 317–331 (2020)
29. O'Loughlin, G., Cullen, S.J., McGoldrick, A., O'Connor, S., Blain, R., O'Malley, S., Warrington, G.D.: Using a wearable camera to increase the accuracy of dietary analysis. Am. J. Preventive Med. **44**(3), 297–301 (2013). https://doi.org/10.1016/j.amepre.2012.11.007. http://www.sciencedirect.com/science/article/pii/S074937971200863X
30. Pu, Q., Gupta, S., Gollakota, S., Patel, S.: Whole-home gesture recognition using wireless signals. In: Proceedings of the 19th Annual International Conference on Mobile Computing & Networking, MobiCom '13, p. 27–38. Association for Computing Machinery, New York (2013). https://doi.org/10.1145/2500423.2500436
31. Ren, W., Ma, O., Ji, H., Liu, X.: Human posture recognition using a hybrid of fuzzy logic and machine learning approaches. IEEE Access **8**, 135628–135639 (2020)
32. Ren, Y., Chen, Y., Chuah, M.C., Yang, J.: Smartphone based user verification leveraging gait recognition for mobile healthcare systems. In: 2013 IEEE International Conference on Sensing, Communications and Networking (SECON), pp. 149–157 (2013)
33. Saadeh, W., Aslam, S.Z., Hina, A., Asghar, F.: A 0.5v ppg-based heart rate and variability detection system. In: 2018 IEEE Biomedical Circuits and Systems Conference (BioCAS), pp. 1–4 (2018)
34. Saidi, H., Labraoui, N., Abba Ari, A.A., Semahi, I., Mamcha, B.R.: Real-time aging friendly fall detection system. In: 2019 6th International Conference on Image and Signal Processing and their Applications (ISPA), pp. 1–6 (2019)
35. Shearwood, C., Williams, C.B., Mellor, P.H., Yates, R.B., Gibbs, M.R.J., Mattingley, A.D.: Levitation of a micromachined rotor for application in a rotating gyroscope. Electron. Lett. **31**(21), 1845–1846 (1995)
36. Song, C., Wang, A., Ren, K., Xu, W.: Eyeveri: A secure and usable approach for smartphone user authentication. In: IEEE INFOCOM 2016-The 35th Annual IEEE International Conference on Computer Communications, pp. 1–9. IEEE (2016)
37. Straczkiewicz, M., James, P., Onnela, J.P.: A systematic review of smartphone-based human activity recognition methods for health research. NPJ Digit. Med. **4**(1), 148 (2021)
38. Sun, M., Fernstrom, J.D., Jia, W., Hackworth, S.A., Yao, N., Li, Y., Li, C., Fernstrom, M.H., Sclabassi, R.J.: A wearable electronic system for objective dietary assessment. J. Am. Diet. Assoc. **110**(1), 45–47 (2010). https://doi.org/10.1016/j.jada.2009.10.013. http://www.sciencedirect.com/science/article/pii/S0002822309016897

39. Sun, F., Mao, C., Fan, X., Li, Y.: Accelerometer-based speed-adaptive gait authentication method for wearable iot devices. IEEE Internet Things J. **6**(1), 820–830 (2018)
40. Tran, K.M., Johnson, R.K., Soultanakis, R.P., Matthews, D.E.: In-person vs telephone-administered multiple-pass 24-hour recalls in women: validation with doubly labeled water. J. Am. Diet. Assoc. **100**(7), 777–783 (2000)
41. Wang, Y., Liu, J., Chen, Y., Gruteser, M., Yang, J., Liu, H.: E-eyes: device-free location-oriented activity identification using fine-grained wifi signatures. In: Proceedings of the 20th Annual International Conference on Mobile Computing & Networking, pp. 617–628 (2014)
42. Wang, X., Yang, C., Mao, S.: Phasebeat: exploiting csi phase data for vital sign monitoring with commodity wifi devices. In: 2017 IEEE 37th International Conference on Distributed Computing Systems (ICDCS), pp. 1230–1239 (2017)
43. Wang, F., Feng, J., Zhao, Y., Zhang, X., Zhang, S., Han, J.: Joint activity recognition and indoor localization with wifi fingerprints. IEEE Access **7**, 80058–80068 (2019)
44. Yang, D., Huangfu, J.: Improving activity recognition for multiple-node wireless sensor network system based on compressed sensing. Int. J. Sensor Netw. **34**(3), 162–171 (2020)
45. Zeng, Y., Pathak, P.H., Yang, Z., Mohapatra, P.: Poster abstract: human tracking and activity monitoring using 60 ghz mmwave. In: 2016 15th ACM/IEEE International Conference on Information Processing in Sensor Networks (IPSN), pp. 1–2 (2016)
46. Zhang, W., Ni, H., He, M., Liu, J., Wang, Z., Zhou, X.: Ifc: Your invisible fitness coach based on csi sensing. In: 2019 IEEE SmartWorld, Ubiquitous Intelligence & Computing, Advanced & Trusted Computing, Scalable Computing & Communications, Cloud & Big Data Computing, Internet of People and Smart City Innovation (SmartWorld/SCALCOM/UIC/ATC/CBDCom/IOP/SCI), pp. 1011–1018. IEEE (2019)
47. Zhang, J., Wu, F., Wei, B., Zhang, Q., Huang, H., Shah, S.W., Cheng, J.: Data augmentation and dense-lstm for human activity recognition using wifi signal. IEEE Internet Things J. **8**(6), 4628–4641 (2020)
48. Zhou, H., Gao, Y., Liu, W., Jiang, Y., Dong, W.: Posture tracking meets fitness coaching: A two-phase optimization approach with wearable devices. In: 2020 IEEE 17th International Conference on Mobile Ad Hoc and Sensor Systems (MASS), pp. 524–532. IEEE (2020)
49. Zhu, F., Bosch, M., Boushey, C.J., Delp, E.J.: An image analysis system for dietary assessment and evaluation. In: 2010 IEEE International Conference on Image Processing, pp. 1853–1856 (2010)
50. Zhu, Y., Wang, D., Zhao, R., Zhang, Q., Huang, A.: Fitassist: Virtual fitness assistant based on wifi. In: Proceedings of the 16th EAI International Conference on Mobile and Ubiquitous Systems: Computing, Networking and Services, pp. 328–337 (2019)

Chapter 2
Contactless Activity Identification Using Commodity WiFi

Activity monitoring in home environments has become increasingly crucial for elder care, well-being management, and latchkey child safety. However, traditional approaches require expensive wearable sensors or specialized hardware installations, which can be intrusive and uncomfortable. To address this issue, this chapter presents a low-cost system for device-free and location-oriented activity identification at home using existing WiFi access points and devices. The system leverages the complex web of WiFi links and fine-grained channel state information that can be extracted from them to identify both in-place activities and walking movements by comparing them against signal profiles. The construction of signal profiles can be semi-supervised and adaptively updated to account for the movement of mobile devices and signal calibration. Experimental evaluation in two apartments of different sizes demonstrates that our approach achieves a high average true positive rate for distinguishing a set of in-place and walking activities with only a single WiFi access point. Furthermore, the prototype also indicates that the system can work with a wider signal band (802.11ac) with even higher accuracy, making it a promising alternative to traditional approaches for activity monitoring in home environments.

The reminder of this chapter is organized as follows: We present the research background in Sect. 2.1 and discuss related work in Sect. 2.2. Next, we provide the design of the CSI-based activity identification system in Sect. 2.3. In Sect. 2.4, we elaborate the designed activity recognition schemes. Then, we describe the system implementation in Sect. 2.5. In Sect. 2.6, we perform the evaluation of our system in real environments. Finally, we provide a discussion and conclude our work in Sect. 2.7.

X. Guo et al., *Mobile Technologies for Smart Healthcare System Design*,
Wireless Networks, https://doi.org/10.1007/978-3-031-57345-3_2

2.1 Background

There exist a broad range of applications that benefit from higher-level contextual information—an understanding of activities that persons are engaged in, not just their positions inside a coordinate system. For example, activity recognition is an essential part of a trend towards the quantified self. By tracking a sequence of meaningful activities and generating statistics for a person, it is possible to monitor well-being and suggest behavioral changes that improve health. Such activity tracking is arguably even more compelling for children and the elderly. In aging-in-place settings, it can be helpful to understand whether established routines are still followed since the absence of usual activities can be an important indicator for detecting falls and other situations needing immediate attentions. The challenge in activity recognition for these applications lies in finding solutions that can provide sufficiently accurate tracking and recognition with minimal infrastructure requirements and without the need to carry a dedicated device. Existing activity recognition solutions [13, 16, 19, 30, 38] primarily rely on dedicated tracking sensors worn by people or cameras, motion sensors, etc. installed in surroundings [16, 28]. These solutions require either significant infrastructure installation or diligent usage of the wearable device. More generally, some activities that are tied to particular places can also be inferred from location systems [4, 40], either device-based or device-free, but these systems cannot distinguish multiple activities that occur in the same place. Device-free systems do not require persons to carry any devices, but they require a dense placement of multiple sensors to create a mesh of wireless links inside the area of interest. Perhaps most related to our work is the effort to use detailed physical layer measurements such as Doppler shifts from one single wireless monitor to detect people's movement, location, and even gestures. The granularity of the monitoring ranges from coarser movements (such as Wi-Vi [1]) to fine-grained gestures (such as WiSee [21] and WiTrack [2]). However, these systems all have been prototyped with USRP software radios and require a specialized receiver that extracts carrier wave features that are not reported in current WiFi systems. In addition, activity identification differs from gesture recognition in that the system needs to identify a more loosely defined series of motions over a period of time rather than a single well-defined body movement. For example, an activity such as cooking includes several movements to fetch, prepare, and mix ingredients that are not always exactly the same and do not necessarily occur in the same sequence, making it difficult to detect with gesture recognition techniques that are designed for precise single motions such as punching a boxing bag.

This chapter explores a novel development in the design space and demonstrates that device-free location-oriented activity recognition is possible by (1) using the existing channel state information provided by IEEE 802.11n devices and (2) using relatively few wireless links, such as those to existing in-home WiFi devices. The system exploits the trend to wider bandwidths (e.g., 802.11ac), and in particular, the more fine-grained channel state information that is being tracked in MIMO communications. Whereas traditional received signal strength (RSS) measurements are a single quantity per packet that represents signal-to-interference-plus-noise ratio (SINR) over the channel bandwidth, channel state information contains amplitude and phase measurements separately for each OFDM subcarrier. Due to the slight frequency delta, separate subcarriers experience different multipath fading. While such effects are often averaged out, when looking at a single average RSS measurement, the individual subcarrier measurements are more likely to change when small movements have altered the multipath environment. This essentially means that our system will not just detect obstructions on the direct path but can also take advantage of the rich web of reflected rays to cover a space. This makes it possible to operate with a single access point and a small set of stationary WiFi devices, which likely already exist or will exist soon in many buildings.

The contributions of this chapter are summarized as follows: In this chapter, we demonstrate the utilization of channel state information (CSI) obtained from off-the-shelf 802.11n devices to identify and differentiate in-place activities within a home, using a smaller set of transmitting devices compared to previous device-free localization solutions. Moreover, we develop a monitoring framework that operates on a single WiFi access point (AP) and its connected devices, employing profile matching algorithms to compare amplitude profiles with known activities. Furthermore, we investigate dynamic profile construction, enabling adaptive updates to accommodate device movement or replacement and daily profile calibration. Through extensive experiments conducted in two different-sized apartments, we establish that a single AP with 3 connected devices can accurately distinguish 8 walking activities between rooms (20 rounds each), 9 daily activities (50 rounds each), and over 100 rounds of other activities with an average detection rate exceeding 96% and an average false positive rate below 1%. Even with just one device, the detection rate remains around 92% with a similar false positive rate. In addition, we demonstrate how the trend towards wider channels, such as 802.11ac, enhances recognition by allowing measurements over additional subcarriers.

2.2 Related Work

There has been active work in using dedicated sensors for activity recognition [13, 16, 19, 20, 28, 30, 36, 38]. Sensors can be either attached to a person's body [13], or placed on target objects with which people interact [30]. For example, an accelerometer is attached on a human body to detect falls in Philips Lifeline [20], whereas a motion sensor is attached to a door to detect movement in GrandCare [28]. Another example of using wearable sensor is case of the acoustic sensor used in BodyScop for classifying activities, such as eating and coughing [38]. Vision based systems [16], such as Leap Motion (https://www.leapmotion.com) and Kinect [19], can be used to track user movements and gestures. These dedicated sensors can achieve fine-grained activity recognition. However, they need the installation and maintenance of dedicated sensors which usually entail high costs and are thus not scalable.

Another body of related work is indoor localization systems which can be extended to activity recognition [3–6, 8, 12, 14, 17, 18, 26, 31, 33, 34, 37, 39]. These systems localize a wireless emitter using Received Signal Strength (RSS) [3–5, 8, 14, 18, 34, 37, 39], OFDM channel state information [26], antenna arrays [12, 33], RFID tags [31], rotating anchors [6], or visible LED lights [17]. These systems provide various accuracy ranging from several meters (e.g., RSS-based) to sub-meter but require people to carry a wireless emitter. This can be intrusive and problematic, especially for elderlies, with memory loss, who often forget to carry such devices. . Furthermore, they need the support of wireless infrastructure, either lightweight devices such as re-use multiple access points if available [4, 8, 18] or costly specialized devices, such as antenna arrays [12, 33]. The infrastructural cost of these systems thus prevents their large scale deployment.

The radio tomography imaging (RTI) [32, 41] and device-free passive (DfP) localization [15, 25, 35, 40], like our system, do not require a device be attached to or carried by the user. The state of art RTI requires tens or hundreds of wireless sensors to achieve sub-meter accuracy, while DfP localization [15, 25] with four WiFi APs has an accuracy of several meters. Several works [10, 27] propose to distinguish some basic activities such as walking, crawling, standing and lying based on RSS using a set of receivers or USRP SDR devices. These systems are either impractical for roaming deployment or not accurate enough for fine-grained activity recognition.

Recent work in using a single wireless monitor to detect human movement or location [1, 2, 21] can be used for activity recognition as well. The granularity of the activity can be inferred from these systems is either modest (such as Wi-Vi [1]) or fine-grained (such as WiSee [21] and WiTrack [2]). However, these systems all require specialized WiFi monitors (e.g., USRP) for extracting the carrier wave. In contrast, we use an off-the-shelf WiFi device for activity recognition. Our method can provide fine-grained activity recognition by re-using existing home WiFi network and thus has much higher scalability for wide deployment. Furthermore, different from WiSee that focuses on recognizing well-defined, quick gestures, our work aims to discriminate loosely defined daily activities that involve a series of body movements over a certain period of time. In recognizing such loosely defined daily activities, we find that channel characteristics, such as the statistical distribution and time series, are more suitable for distinguishing between activities lasting a certain period of time than quick gestures.

2.3 CSI-based Activity Identification System Design

2.3.1 Feasibility of Using CSI for Activity Identification

This study aims to leverage two notable trends in the realm of WiFi usage. Firstly, the application of WiFi has broadened, transitioning from merely facilitating internet connectivity for laptops to connecting a host of smart devices, such as televisions, game consoles, surveillance cameras, refrigerators, and loudspeakers to home networks and the internet. This has resulted in an augmented number of WiFi links within households, a subset of which employ continuous beaconing. Secondly, WiFi radios now offer more granular channel measurements across larger bandwidths. The advent of 802.11n MIMO systems necessitated more refined tracking of channel state information by radios. In its standard 20 MHz channel, 802.11n radios are capable of gauging the amplitude and phase for each of the 52 orthogonal frequency-division multiplexing (OFDM) subcarriers. Furthermore, when operating with 40 MHz channels, measurements can be obtained for 128 subcarriers. The emerging IEEE 802.11ac standard is even anticipated to support broader bandwidths. These measurements essentially facilitate the estimation of the channel frequency response, contrasting with the traditional received signal strength (RSS) which provided merely a single value per packet, typically a SINR reading averaged over the entire channel bandwidth.

Measuring the channel frequency response has important implications for detecting and differentiating minute movements. Inside buildings, signal propagation is dominated by multipath, with the received signal amplitude (or strength) resulting from combining amplitudes of signals arriving over many different paths (scattered from and reflected off different objects). Since the individual signals can constructively or deconstructively, combine based on their individual phase shifts, this effect can lead to large differences in the combined amplitude, which is commonly known as small-scale fading. A small change in frequency, however, can have a large effect on the combined signal. The amount of frequency change for a signal amplitude to become uncorrelated with its previous value is also known as the coherence bandwidth and can be estimated as $B_c = \frac{1}{D}$, where D is the delay spread of the arriving multipath signals. Interestingly, the width of an OFDM subcarrier is chosen to match this coherence bandwidth to simplify receiver design. This means that amplitude measurements on each subcarrier will provide many uncorrelated combinations of the received multipath components, which increase the likelihood that some are affected by a small movement. A single RSS measurement over the signal bandwidth, in comparison, averages out many of these detailed small scale fading effects.

Figure 2.1 shows a motivational experiment where two different activities were conducted in the same location: talking on the phone and washing dishes. The histograms of RSS readings collected for both of these activities show relatively little difference. The histograms of CSI amplitudes (quantized to 20 bins) for a specific subcarrier, however, show very distinct distributions that can be used to clearly distinguish these different movements in the same location. The insight is that since an activity involves a series of body movements during a certain period of time, the distribution of CSI amplitudes is a desirable channel statistic that can capture unique characteristics of activities in both time and frequency domains.

With more WiFi devices in homes and the ability to measure small changes in multipath rays, our intuition suggests that it might be possible to track activities and movements around a home with only this existing infrastructure. Device-free localization and activity recognition requires that at least one measurable RF ray

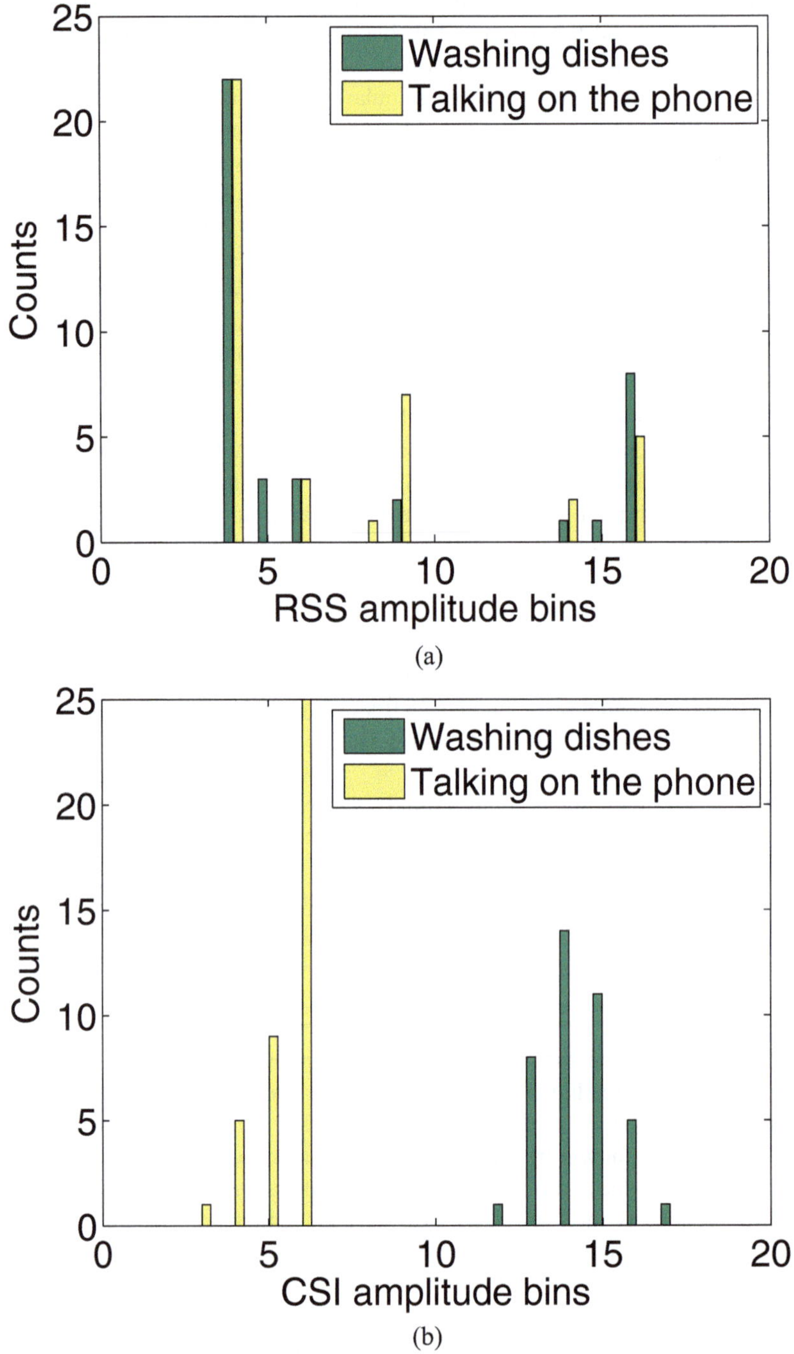

Fig. 2.1 Histograms of RSS amplitude and CSI amplitude of a particular subcarrier for two different in-place activities at the same position: washing dishes and talking on the phone nearby the sink. (**a**) 1-bedroom apartment. (**b**) 2-bedroom apartment

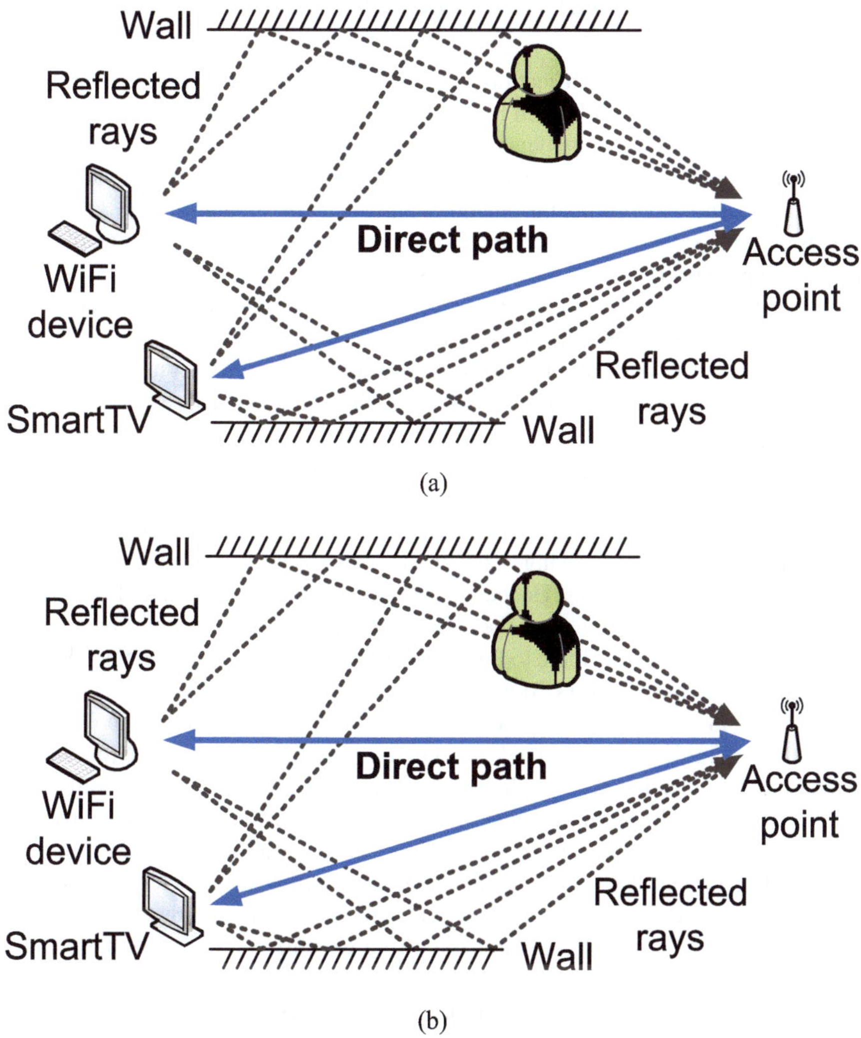

Fig. 2.2 CSI takes the advantage of multipath effects and captures the detailed changes on different subcarriers. (**a**) Existing work: link-centric using RSS. (**b**) Illustration of reflected rays

travels through any location of interest, because the presence or movement of a human body at this position would only alter the propagation of these rays. Earlier device free localization system have therefore blanketed spaces with multiple transceivers to create a fine mesh of measurable direct links. As illustrated in Fig. 2.2a and b, such a measurable mesh can now also be created by all the multipath rays from only a handful of WiFi devices instead of requiring many additional devices.

2.3.2 Contactless Activity Identification System Design

Developing a system that can accurately recognize activities at an access point using CSI measurements from a limited number of WiFi links presents many challenges. For example, one crucial challenge is ensuring the uniqueness and robustness of activity profiles. CSI measurements are susceptible to signal interferences, user movements, and environmental changes, making it necessary for the system to match activity signatures or features to measurements that are both resilient to noise in real-world WiFi device readings and distinct enough to correspond to specific activities. Another significant challenge is achieving algorithm generality. Different activities require different types of information for successful differentiation. For instance, one activity may involve walking between rooms, resulting in CSI measurements without obvious patterns, while another activity like washing dishes in the kitchen entails repetitive gestures, leading to CSI measurements with repetitive patterns. These varying characteristics demand an algorithm that can handle and identify activities with diverse signal patterns. Additionally, profile generation poses a challenge, particularly during system installation or when significant environmental changes occur. In such cases, there may be a lack of existing profiles for activities. Hence, the system should have the capability to assist in profile generation, alleviating the effort required for this process. Overcoming these challenges will contribute to the development of a robust and efficient activity recognition system based on CSI measurements.

The basic idea of our system is to match CSI patterns against activity profiles. As illustrated in Fig. 2.3, the system takes as input time-series amplitude measurements, which can be collected at a single access point with off-the-shelf hardware (e.g., Intel 5300 NIC). The amplitude measurements are available for each subcarrier on a link and are collected over several links to mostly stationary devices (such as home entertainment devices or appliances). We discuss later on how the system might be extended to also use mobile devices when they do not move. The system can take advantage of CSI measurements from existing traffic across these links. If insufficient network traffic is available, the system might also generate periodic traffic for measurement purposes. This data is then preprocessed to remove outliers via a low-pass filter and to filter out artifacts introduces by rate adaptation, where the radios switch to different modulation and coding schemes.

The core components of our system, are the *Activity Identification* and the *Profile Construction and Updating*. Activity identification encompasses two different activity matching approaches to address the generality challenge. The system distinguishes between walking activities and in-place activities. In general, a walking activity causes significant pattern changes of the CSI amplitude over time, since it involves significant body movements and location changes. An in-place activity (such as watching TV on a sofa) only involves relative smaller body movements and will not cause significant amplitude changes but present certain repetitive patterns. It thus first applies a moving variance thresholding technique to discriminate the two types of activities. The cumulative moving variance across all subcarriers can be expected to be greater for walking activities than in-place activities. Moreover,

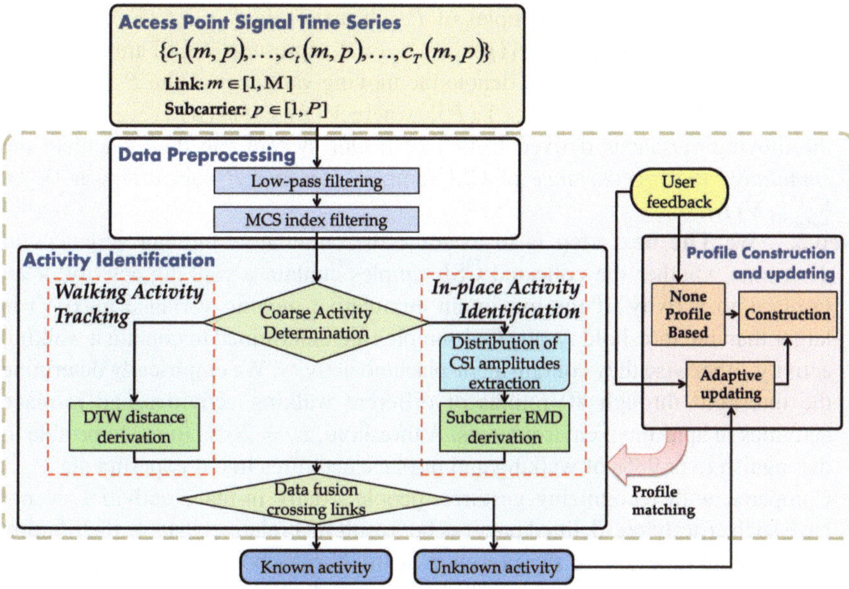

Fig. 2.3 System flow of activity recognition using CSI

our system leverages the moving variance to segment the long-term CSI trace. Since the trace often contains multiple different activities over time, moving variance is used to determine the start and end of individual activities.

2.4 Activity Identification Categories

In this section, we first describe *Coarse-grained Activity Determination*. We then present *In-place Activity Identification* and *Walking Activity Tracking* components in our system. And we also discuss how our system can benefit from wider signal bandwidths using 802.11ac.

2.4.1 Coarse-grained Activity Determination

Since various activities cause different degrees of signal changes, we apply the *moving variance* on top of the CSI measurements to capture this difference and determine the category of the activity. In particular, a large moving variance indicates the presence of a walking activity whereas a small moving variance represents the presence of an in-place activity or no activity at all. The detailed steps are presented as follows:

Step 1. We denote the CSI samples of P subcarriers as $C = \{C(1), \ldots, C(p), \ldots, C(P)\}$, where $C(p) = [c_1(p), \ldots, c_T(p)]'$ represents T CSI amplitudes on the pth subcarrier. We further denote the moving variances of the P subcarriers as $V = \{V(1), \ldots, V(p), \ldots, V(P)\}$, where $V(p) = [v_1(p), \ldots, v_T(p)]$ are the moving variances derived from $C(P)$. Our system can then calculate the *cumulative moving variance* of CSI samples crossing P subcarriers as $\mathcal{V} = \sum_{p=1}^{P} V(p)$.

Step 2. We **The next step is to** examine the cumulative moving variances to determine whether the collected CSI samples contain a walking activity or an in-place/no activity. If the maximum cumulative moving variance $\max(\mathcal{V})$ is larger than the threshold τ_v, the CSI samples are determined to contain a walking activity, otherwise they contain an in-place/no activity. We empirically determine the threshold through 40 rounds of different walking activities and in-place activities in apartment environments. A threshold, $\tau_v = 20$, is found to be able to distinguish over 98% of walking and in-place activities in our experiments.

Compared with recognizing gestures, people's daily in-place activities do not have such strictly pre-defined patterns but result in a relatively stable distribution of CSI amplitude due to the presence of the human body and loosely defined body motions. In our system, segmentation is first performed in the task of Coarse Activity Determination by examining the CSI variance in the collected trace. Note that Coarse Activity Determination can be also used to identify the starting and ending of both walking activities and in-place activities, since walking activities often separate in-place activities. If the segmented CSI trace belongs to an in-place activity, we will further use the EMD technique [24] to compare the distribution of CSI amplitudes in a sliding time window with in-place activity profiles to identify different activities within this trace. If the segmented CSI trace is recognized as a walking activity, we will further identify the walking trajectory or the passing of doorways.

2.4.2 *In-place Activity Identification*

2.4.2.1 Activity Characteristics Analysis

We find that an in-place activity results in a relatively stable distribution of CSI amplitude due to the presence of the human body and (possibly) repetitive body movement over time. Furthermore, different in-place activities cause different distributions of CSI amplitude as the location and/or the repetitive body movement patterns and the posture of the human body are different for different in-place activities. We illustrate the similarity of the CSI amplitude distribution for the same activity, and the difference of the CSI amplitude distribution for two different in-place activities (i.e., cooking in a kitchen and sleeping on a bed) at a particular subcarrier (subcarrier 12) in Figs. 2.4 and 2.5. We observe that the CSI amplitude distributions are similar for the same activity at different rounds, but distinctive for

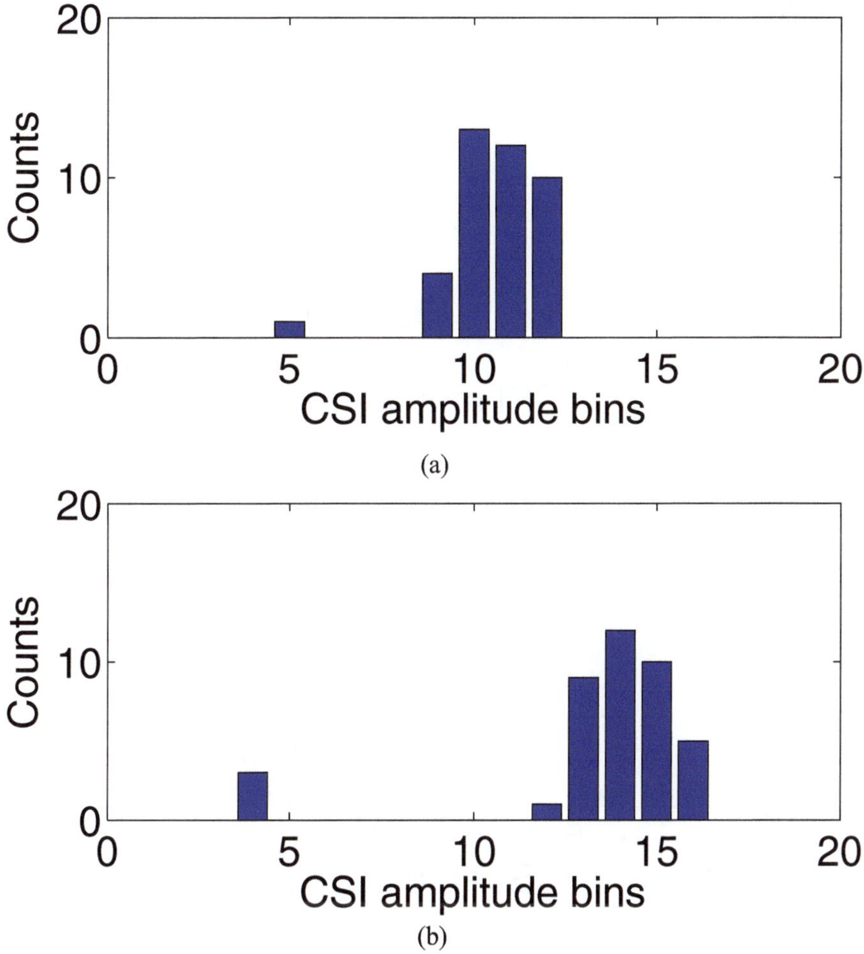

Fig. 2.4 Histogram of CSI amplitudes on a particular subcarrier for cooking and sleeping (round 1). (**a**) Cooking, round 1. (**b**) Sleeping, round 1

different activities. This important observation inspires us to exploit the distribution of CSI amplitude to distinguish different in-place activities and shows that a particular in-place activity can be identified by comparing against known profiles.

2.4.2.2 In-place Activity Classifier Design

Based on the characteristics of the in-place activities, we employ the earth mover's distance (EMD) technique, which is a well-known approach for evaluating the similarity between two probability distributions. The EMD calculates the minimal cost to transform one distribution into the other. Our classifier seeks to compare the

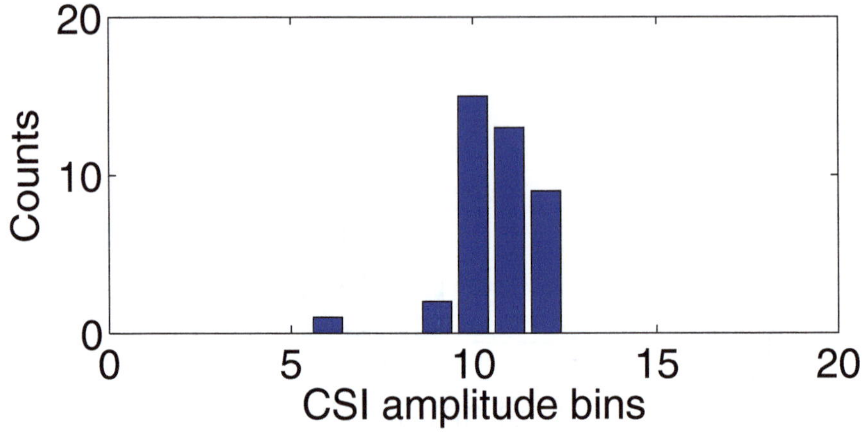

(a)

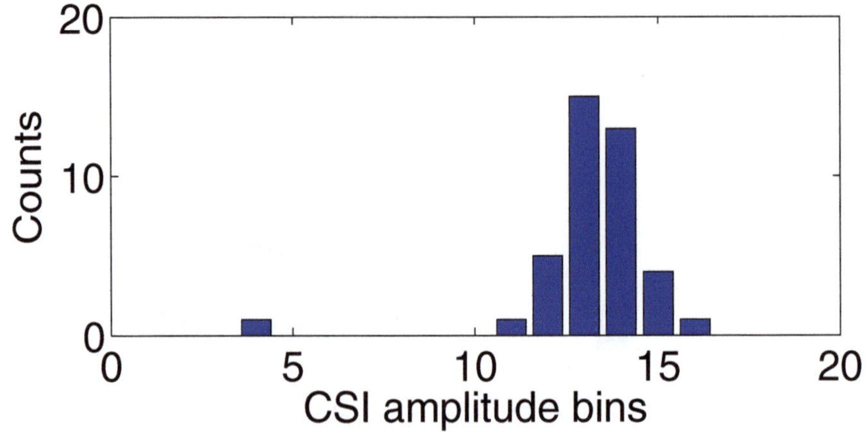

(b)

Fig. 2.5 Histogram of CSI amplitudes on a particular subcarrier for cooking and sleeping (round 2). (**a**) Cooking, round 2. (**b**) Sleeping, round 2

distribution of the testing CSI measurements to those of the known in-place activity profiles by using the EMD metric. CSI measurements being tested are identified to contain a known activity when the resulted minimal cost (i.e., minimal EMD distance) is small enough.

Specifically, at run time, our system first identifies the testing CSI measurements as a *candidate* of a particular known in-place activity if the EMD distance from the candidate to the known in-place activity is the minimum among the EMD distances to all known activities stored in the CSI profiles. Then our system further confirms the candidate undergoing in-place activity by comparing the resulted minimal EMD distance to a threshold, which can be empirically determined in the profile construction. The candidate known in-place activity is confirmed if the minimal EMD distance is less than the threshold, otherwise, it will be identified as an unknown activity. An alternate way to determine whether the testing CSI measurements correspond to a known activity or not is to use an outlier detection method, such as the median absolute deviation (MAD) [23], to examine whether the resultant minimum EMD distance is within a range. To determine the range, an EMD distance pool containing the minimal EMD distances of previous successfully identified activities is needed in the profiles. We note that our system can also recognize the same in-place activities occurring in different locations by comparing the testing CSI measurements to a set of CSI profiles constructed when the same activities occur in different locations. In this case, the profile for an activity is a set of CSI profiles instead of a single CSI profile, and the testing CSI measurements are determined to contain the activity if it has the minimum EMD distance to any of the CSI profiles belonging to the activity profile.

2.4.3 Tracking Walking Activity

2.4.3.1 Walking Activity Characteristics

We find that the CSI collected from walking activities is changing constantly over time due to body movement and change of locations. In particular, Figs. 2.6 and 2.7 presents CSI amplitude of each subcarrier versus the packet index (i.e., time series) for two different walking paths in two experimental runs. We observe that the CSI measurements exhibit similar changing patterns for the same trajectory in different rounds, whereas the changes of CSI measurements over time are different for different trajectories. This observation indicates that the CSI pattern is dominated by the unique path of each walking activity.

Furthermore, since there are always in-place activities before and after a walking activity, ideally we can identify the walking activity by identifying the in-place activities at both ends. However, the starting and ending points of the walking activity can be anywhere inside the space. It is possible that the two endpoints are not that meaningful and thus no such in-place activity profiles are constructed. To tackle this problem, we further build the CSI measurement profile when the person passes through doorways. Since, in general, a person must pass through a door way when walking from one room to another, they can be utilized to facilitate walking activity tracking. By identifying the doorway the person moves through, our system can determine a walking activity in high level without requiring extensive profiling of paths that have less meaningful starting and ending locations.

2.4.3.2 Walking Activity Discrimination

Walking Path Discrimination Since people may walk at different speeds for the same trajectory, we use Dynamic Time Warping (DTW) [22] to align the

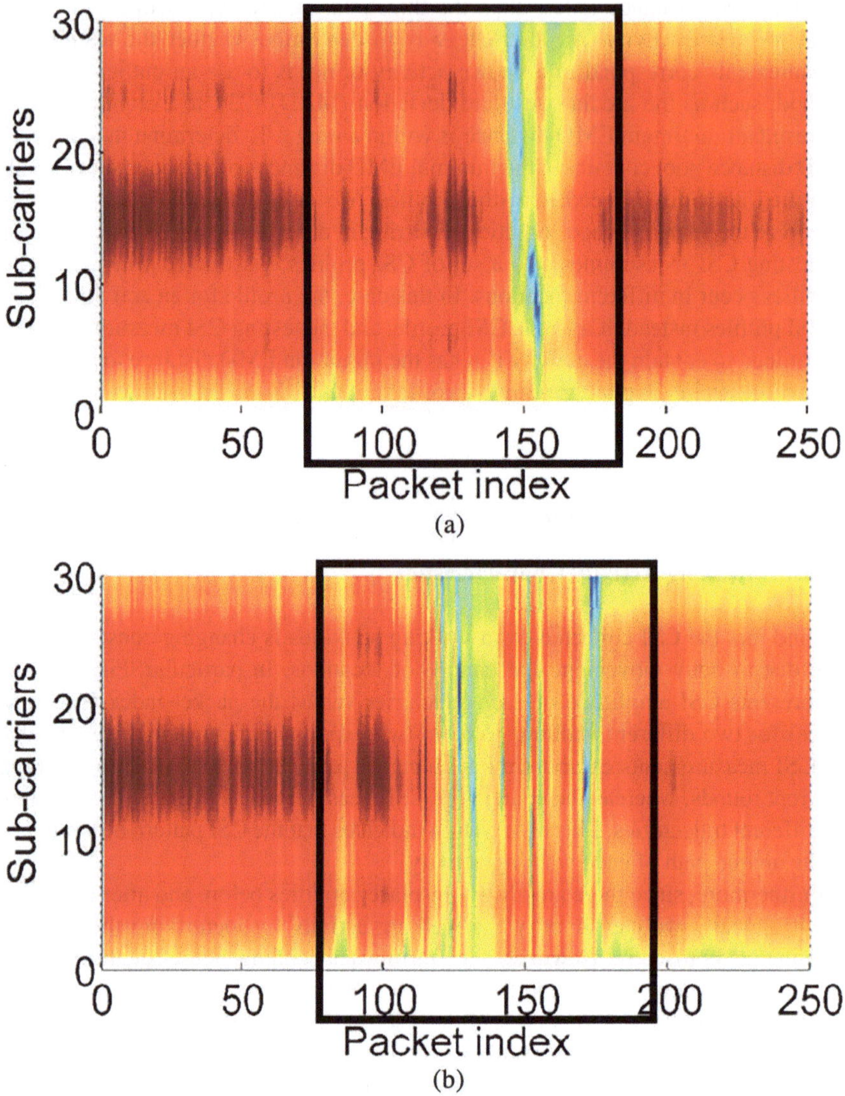

Fig. 2.6 Similar CSI time series pattern for same walking trajectory (round 1). (**a**) Trajectory 1, round 1. (**b**) Trajectory 2, round 1

testing CSI measurements to those from known activities in the profile. We then identify the activity based on the similarity measures using DTW. DTW stretches and compresses required parts to allow a proper comparison between two data sequences. This is useful to match CSI samples from different walking speeds in real-world scenarios. In our system, CSI measurements are in a format that reports

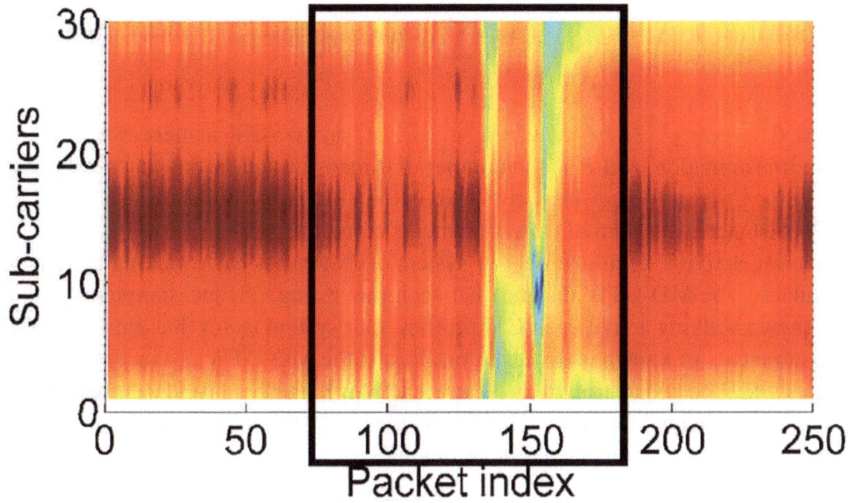

(a)

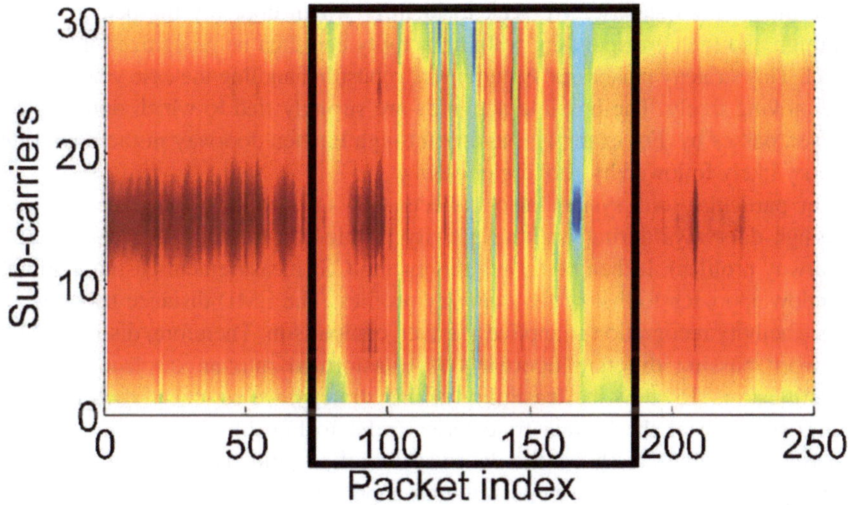

(b)

Fig. 2.7 Similar CSI time series pattern for same walking trajectory (round 2). (**a**) Trajectory 1, round 2. (**b**) Trajectory 2, round 2

the channel metrics for multiple subcarrier groups (e.g., 30 subcarriers). To perform multi-dimensional sequence alignment, our system employs Multi-Dimensional Dynamic Time Warping (MD-DTW) [29], in which the vector norm is utilized to calculate the distance matrix according to:

$$d(c_i, c'_j) = \sum_{p=1}^{P} (c_i(p) - c'_j(p))^2, \tag{2.1}$$

where $C = c_1, c_2, \ldots, c_T$ and $C'=c'_1, c'_2, \ldots, c'_T$ are two CSI sequences for walking path discrimination, and P is the number of dimensions of the sequence data (with P=30 for CSI sample). A least cost path is found through this matrix and the MD-DTW distance is the sum of matrix elements along the path.

During activity identification, our system distinguishes each walking activity by calculating the MD-DTW distance between the testing CSI measurements and all the known walking activities in CSI profiles. Our system stores the segment of CSI measurements of known activities in profiles. If the MD-DTW distance is less than a threshold (i.e., considering it as a known activity), we then take the corresponding CSI measurements labeled in the CSI profiles with the minimum distance as the activity identified for the testing measurements.

Doorway Discrimination Doorway discrimination is used to handle the case where the testing CSI measurements are unknown after our attempt to match them with the profile database. We seek to identify which doorway the person passes through and the corresponding walking activity can then be recognized in a high-level. This strategy makes our system more robust in handling the case when people are moving freely. The possible activities are strongly tied to which doorway the person passes by. For example, passing through kitchen doorway in the noon time is very likely followed by cooking or eating.

In particular, our system also collects CSI for profiling when people pass through doorways during walking activity profile construction (i.e., constructing doorway profiles). It then compares the testing CSI measurements using a sliding window approach to that of the doorway profiles. The EMD distance used the in-place activity recognition is applied for such comparison. Therefore, distinguishing between passing different doorways is transformed into an in-place activities identification. To show the feasibility of this strategy, we conduct experiments 20 times for each of the 8 walk trajectories (refer to Fig. 2.8) in two different-size apartments. Table 2.1 shows the doorway detection ratio (DR) of each trajectory corresponding to the doorway passed. Our approach achieves an average detection accuracy of over 96.25%, which is sufficient as a supplement to walking trajectory discrimination.

2.5 Activity Identification Sensing System Implementation

2.5.1 Activity Profile Construction

In our system, we collect the CSI measurements of typical activities for profile construction. In particular, we use the distribution of CSI amplitude to profile in-

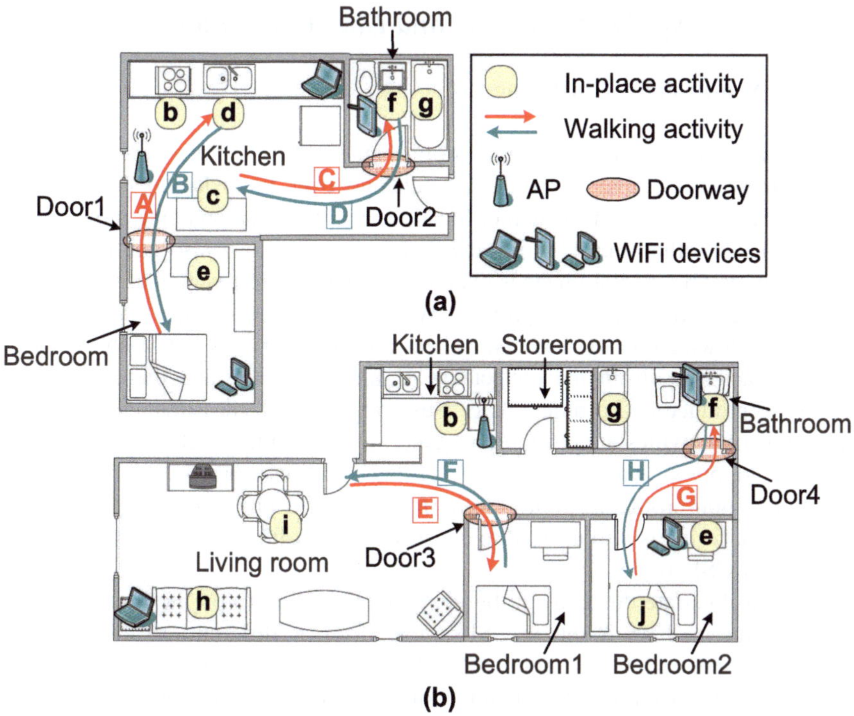

Fig. 2.8 Experimental setups and the illustration of activities in two different-size apartments: (**a**) one-bedroom apartment and (**b**) two-bedroom apartment

Table 2.1 Doorway detection accuracy

1-BR Apt.	Bedroom↔Kitchen	Kitchen↔Bathroom
DR	1	0.975
2-BR Apt.	Outside↔Bedroom1	Bedroom2↔Bathroom
DR	1	0.875

place activities and the sequence of CSI amplitude for walking activities. If multiple WiFi devices are available, the profile is constructed by using each WiFi device. Additionally, we build a profile for "empty room" (i.e., no one inside the room), which is a special case of an in-place activity. When constructing profiles, it is possible that the profile of an activity from a particular WiFi device is similar to the profile of "empty room" when the activity is very far away from that device.

2.5.2 *Non-profiling Clustering and Data Calibration*

2.5.2.1 Non-profiling Clustering

After profile construction, the activity profiles may still change due to many factors. For example, the activity profiles may change over time due to the involved WiFi device being moved to another location, e.g., the desktop being moved from one room to another. Furthermore, the activity profiles may also get affected by day-to-day environmental changes. Therefore, our system requires a method that can adaptively update activity profiles. We design a process called *non-profiling clustering*, in which the system first utilizes a semi-supervised approach to cluster the daily activities from the collected CSI measurements, and then label each activity to produce CSI profiles. After clustering, the CSI measurements from the same type of activities are clustered together. Once significant changes of profiles are detected, our system utilizes users' feedback (i.e., user labels each new cluster returned by non-profile clustering) to perform adaptive profile updating. The non-profiling clustering is also utilized to construct CSI profiles when our system starts without any CSI profile.

We next illustrate this strategy by applying clustering to profile in-place activities. Assume we have R sets of CSI samples from K different unknown activity instances, where each CSI sample set C^r, $1 \leq r \leq R$, corresponds to one particular activity instance with a certain number of CSI samples. Here we exploit the K-Means clustering technique to discriminate different activity instances based on the EMD between CSI samples.

In order to utilize EMD for clustering, we first calculate the EMD between any particular CSI sample set C^r and all the sample sets (including C^r itself). We then obtain R EMD vectors of length R, i.e., $E^r = \left[E(C^r, C^1), \cdots, E(C^r, C^R)\right]$. Next, the K-means algorithm searches for K appropriate clusters, i.e., $S = s_1, \cdots, s_K$, satisfying the following equation:

$$\arg\min_{S} \sum_{k=1}^{K} \sum_{E^r \in s_k} |E^r - \mu_k|^2, \tag{2.2}$$

where μ_k is the mean value of the EMD vectors in s_k. Equation (2.2) searches for K appropriate clusters S that minimizes the variances of the CSI vectors C^r in each cluster.

Table 2.2 shows the results of clustering based on 400 CSI sample sets involving 8 activity instances, where each set contains 40 CSI samples. Most of the activities can be differentiated from each other with the detection ratio as high as over 84% and an acceptable false positive rate, except for the two activities of brushing and bathing in the bathroom due to the small differences in their corresponding CSI patterns, which cannot be differentiated by clustering.

With the relationship between the activity instances and the clusters S, the CSI sample sets correctly classified are used to create new activity profiles. Furthermore,

Table 2.2 Results of activity identification using clustering without profiles

Test	Empty s_1	Cook. s_2	Eat. s_3	Wash. s_4	Study. s_5	Brush. s_6	Bath. s_7	Other s_8
DR	1	0.98	0.88	0.84	0.92	0.66	0.46	0.94
FPR	0.06	0	0.15	0.09	0	0.45	0.43	0.10

if the profile for a particular activity instance already exists, the system adaptively determines whether to update the activity profile through the comparison with the new profile.

2.5.2.2 Improving CSI Reliability Through Data Calibration

Data calibration is used to improve the reliability of the CSI by mitigating the noise presented in the collected CSI samples. The noise sources could be the complicated indoor propagation, the WiFi devices' inner noise (e.g., vibration or ring of devices), etc.

Low-pass Filtering Low-pass filtering aims to remove high frequency noise which is unlikely caused by human activities as human activities usually have a low frequency range. To remove high frequency noises, we adopt the dynamic exponential smoothing filter (DESF) [7], since it is an exponential smoother that changes its smoothing factor dynamically according to previous samples. The DESF can remove high frequency noise and preserve the features affected by human activities in the CSI measurements.

Modulation and Coding Scheme Index Filtering Besides the effects from human activities, we find that the modulation and coding scheme (MCS) index occasionally changes due to the unstable wireless channel in our experiments, could also influence the amplitude of CSI. To get the changing CSI patterns only affected by human activities, we need to remove the CSI measurements affected by a different MCS index (indicates different channel condition) for a pure reflection metric of human activities.

Specifically, MCS index is a specification of the high-throughput (HT) physical layer (PHY) parameter in 802.11n standard [11]. It contains the information of the modulation order (e.g., BPSK, QPSK, 16-QAM, 64-QAM), the forward error correction (FEC) coding rate, etc, for transmitting a packet. Each 802.11n packet header contains a 16-bit MCS index, which can be extracted together with the CSI sample of each packet. In particular, we find that CSI measurements with the MCS index greater than 263 can make CSI measurements relatively stable in empty rooms even though it changes in such a range. Therefore, we filter out the CSI measurements with MCS value less than 263 and keep the rest of them for activity identification.

2.5.3 Data Fusion Crossing Multiple Links

WiFi usage has expanded from providing Internet access to connecting in-home smart devices such as TVs, refrigerators, and loudspeakers. This provides a number of WiFi links to capture an activity simultaneously inside home. Our system thus can exploit a number of WiFi links to improve the activity recognition accuracy based on the basic schemes.

Assume we have L WiFi devices collecting CSI measurements independently and each device has J activity profiles denoted as $\{a^l_1, \ldots, a^l_j, \ldots, a^l_J\}, l = 1, \ldots, L$. The final activity recognition result is the jth activity (profile) that minimizes the weighted summation of the similarities between the collected CSI measurements and the profiles on each WiFi device, i.e.,

$$a^*_j = \arg\min_j \sum_{l=1}^{L} [w^l_j(a^l_0, a^l_j) \times D^l_j], \tag{2.3}$$

where D^l_j is the EMD or DTW distance between the CSI measurements and the jth activity profile on the lth WiFi device; $w^l_j(a^l_0, a^l_j)$ is the normalized weight dominated by the significance of the jth activity on the lth WiFi device, which is defined as follows:

$$w^l_j(a^l_0, a^l_j) = \frac{1 - \mathcal{X}(a^l_0, a^l_j)}{\sum_{l=1}^{L} [1 - \mathcal{X}(a^l_0, a^l_j)]}, \tag{2.4}$$

where a^l_0 denotes the profile for empty room on the lth WiFi device, and $\mathcal{X}(a^l_0, a^l_j)$ is the cross correlation between the profile of the empty room and the jth activity on the lth WiFi device. To reduce the computational complexity, only the CSI measurements having significant difference from the empty room profile will be included in the above calculation.

2.6 System Evaluation Using Commodity WiFi

2.6.1 Experimental Setup

We conduct experiments in an 802.11n WiFi network with three off-the-shelf WiFi devices (i.e., two Lenovo T500 laptops and one Lenovo T61 laptop) connected to a single commercial wireless access point (i.e., Linksys $E2500$) in two apartments. The laptops run Ubuntu 10.04 LTS with the 2.6.36 kernel and are equipped with Intel WiFi Link 5300 cards for measuring CSI [9]. While CSI information is only publicly exposed by modified drivers for several chipsets, e.g., Intel WiFi Link 5300 and Atheros AR9390, it is internally tracked by 802.11 MIMO implementations. We expect more chipsets will expose such information in the near future.

The packet transmission rate is set to 20 pkts/s. How the rate of packet transmission affects the performance will be discussed in Sect. 2.6.3.5. For each packet, we extract CSI for 30 subcarrier groups, which are evenly distributed in the 56 subcarriers of a 20 MHz channel [11].

We conduct experiments in two apartments of different sizes to test the generality of our system. The experimental setups in these two apartments are shown in Fig. 2.8. The smaller one (i.e., one bedroom apartment) has the size of about 23 ×20 ft with one bedroom, one kitchen and one bathroom, whereas the larger one (i.e., two bedroom apartment) is about 24 ×36 ft with two bed rooms, one storeroom, one kitchen, one living room, and one bathroom. It is commonly accepted that the presence of manifold WiFi devices in home environments is highly possible in the near future. To name a few existing applications: smartTVs in living rooms, thermostats in bedrooms, smart-refrigerators in kitchens, and waterproof wireless speakers in bathrooms. In our experiments, one AP and three WiFi devices are placed at each apartment for daily activity monitoring.

A total of 9 typical daily in-place activities and 8 walking activities (passing through 4 door-ways) with different walking speeds are performed by 4 male adults in both apartments. These activities are listed in Table 2.3, and are shown in Fig. 2.8. The yellow circles show the in-place activities, whereas the red/blue lines represent the paths of the walking activities. Due to different conditions in the two apartments (e.g., having a TV in the living room or not), we have chosen slightly different yet still typical in-place activities to perform in the two apartments. Note that we find it is typical for in-place activities to occur at dedicated locations in home environments, for example activities in a kitchen usually just occur in front of the sink or stove, beside the refrigerator, or at the dining table, whereas activities in a living room usually occur on the couch. In our experiments, the profiles were generated in 1 day and testing data was collected over different days. Over the days, one chair was moved to a different room, coffee makers were moved around in

Table 2.3 Codes for in-place and walking activity profiles

Code	In-place activity	Code	Walking activity
a	Empty apartment	A	Bedroom→Kitchen
b	Cooking	B	Kitchen→Bedroom
c	Eating	C	Kitchen→Bathroom
d	Washing dishes	D	Bathroom→Kitchen
e	Studying at a table	E	Outside→Bedroom1
f	Brushing teeth	F	Bedroom1→Outside
g	Taking a bath	G	Bedroom2→Bathroom
h	Watching TV on a sofa	H	Bathroom→Bedroom2
i	Playing video games	O	Other wandering paths
j	Sleeping on a bed		
o	Other activities		

the kitchen and items on tables, such as bowls and bottles, were moved, as usually occurs in daily life. Moreover, we build the profile for the empty room when there is no one at home (i.e., *Empty apartment (a)*). To test the ability of our system on differentiating diverse in-place activities that occur in the same place, we experiment with 4 in-place activities in the one-bedroom apartment: *sleeping on the bed, sitting on the bed, talking besides the sink, and washing dishes near the sink.* Furthermore, the experimenter conducts several in-place and walking activities which are not profiled (i.e., *Other activities (o)*). They are used to evaluate the robustness of our system for recognizing unknown or random activities.

2.6.2 Evaluation Metrics

We use the following metrics to evaluate the performance of our system.

Confusion Matrix The matrix provides a comprehensive overview of the classification results, illustrating the relationship between the actual activities performed by the user and the corresponding activities classified by our system. Each row in the matrix represents a specific activity performed by the user, while each column represents the activity assigned by our system. By examining the cells within the matrix, we can observe the fractions of activity in each row that were classified as the corresponding activity in each column. This detailed representation allows for a thorough analysis and evaluation of the classification performance of our system in relation to the user's actual activities.

True Positive Rate (TPR) True Positive Rate (TPR) for a specific activity, denoted as A, is a fundamental metric that measures the accuracy of the system in correctly identifying instances of activity A among the total instances of activity A performed by the user. It is calculated as the proportion of instances that are accurately recognized as activity A among all instances where activity A was actually performed. By quantifying the TPR for each activity, we gain valuable insights into the system's ability to accurately identify and classify different activities, providing a comprehensive understanding of its performance in capturing the user's actions.

False Positive Rate (FPR) False Positive Rate (FPR) for a specific activity, denoted as A, is a critical metric that evaluates the system's tendency to incorrectly identify instances as activity A when they are actually different activities. It is calculated as the percentage of instances that are mistakenly classified as activity A among all the testing instances that do not belong to activity A. By analyzing the FPR for each activity, we gain valuable insights into the system's specificity and its potential to generate false alarms or misclassifications. Understanding and monitoring the FPR allows us to assess the system's performance in accurately distinguishing between different activities and minimizing false positives, thereby enhancing its overall reliability and usability.

1-bedroom apt.	a	b	c	d	e	f	g	unknown
a: empty	1							0
b: cooking	0	1						0
c: eating	0	0	1					0
d: washing dishes	0	0	0.16	0.84				0
e: studying	0	0	0	0	1			0
f: brushing	0	0	0.06	0	0	0.94		0
g: bathing	0	0	0.02	0	0	0	0.98	0
o: others	0	0	0	0	0	0	0	1

Actual Activity Performed

Identified In-place Activity

(a)

2-bedroom apt.	a	b	f	g	h	i	j	unknown
a: empty	1							0
b: cooking	0	1						0
f: brushing	0	0	1					0
g: bathing	0	0	0	0.96	0	0	0	0.04
h: watching TV	0	0	0	0	1			0
i: gaming	0	0	0	0	0	1		0
j: sleeping	0	0	0	0	0	0	0.88	0.12
o: others	0	0	0	0	0	0	0.05	0.95

Actual Activity Performed

Identified In-place Activity

(b)

Fig. 2.9 Confusion matrix of in-place activity identification in two different apartments. (**a**) 1-bedroom apartment. (**b**) 2-bedroom apartment

2.6.3 Activity Identification with Multiple WiFi Devices

Figure 2.9 plots the confusion matrix for the in-place activities recognition in two apartments with three WiFi devices. In the one-bedroom apartment, 7 different in-place activities (see Fig. 2.9a) were performed (50 rounds for each). Another 100 rounds of different unknown in-place activities (i.e., *others*) are preformed to evaluate the ability of detecting unknown activities. Similarly, in the two-bedroom apartment, 7 different in-place activities as shown in Fig. 2.9b (each one has 50 rounds) and 100 rounds of unknown activities are performed. For the one-bedroom apartment, the average accuracy of identifying in-place activities is 97% with a standard deviation of 5.66% whereas in the two-bedroom apartment, the average accuracy of identifying in-place activities is 97.38% with a standard deviation of 4.31%.

Figures 2.10 and 2.11 plot the confusion matrix for the walking activities identification and doorway passing detection in two apartments. As shown in

Actual Activity Performed

1-bedroom apt.	A	B	C	D	unknown	Door	Door1	Door2	None
A	1	0	0	0	0	Door1	1	0	0
B	0	1	0	0	0				
C	0	0	0.95	0.05	0	Door2	0	0.975	0.025
D	0	0	0	1	0				
O	0	0	0.1	0	0.9	None	0	0	1

Identified Walking Activity & Doorway

Fig. 2.10 Confusion matrix of walking activity identification in 1-bedroom apartment

Actual Activity Performed

2-bedroom apt.	E	F	G	H	unknown	Door	Door3	Door4	None
E	0	0	0	0	0	Door3	1	0	0
F	0.15	0.85	0	0	0				
G	0	0	0.9	0.1	0	Door4	0	0.875	0.125
H	0	0	0	1	0				
O	0.05	0	0	0	0.95	None	0	0	1

Identified Walking Activity & Doorway

Fig. 2.11 Confusion matrix of walking activity identification in 2-bedroom apartment

Fig. 2.8, 4 trajectories for each apartment are performed, and 20 rounds for each trajectory. Similar to that of the in-place activity experiment, we performed 20 rounds of random walking activities (i.e., walking in the apartment but no passing through predefined doorways) in each apartment as *others*. For the one-bedroom apartment, the average accuracy is 97% when identifying these 4 walking activities. Our system can also achieve high accuracy of detecting doorway passing with an average accuracy of 99.17%. For the two-bedroom apartment, the average accuracy of identifying walking activities is 94%, and the passing doorway can be detected with an accuracy of 95.83%. The above results show that the system can distinguish a set of in-place activities and walking activities with high accuracy by using only a single WiFi access point in two apartments of different size. Our system can thus have potential to support lots of emerging applications such as elder care, well-being management, and latchkey child safety.

2.6.3.1 System Robustness Validation

We next evaluate the robustness of our system by studying the false positive rates (FPRs) of identifying different activities in two apartments. Figures 2.12b and 2.13b show that overall the designed system has very low false positive rates

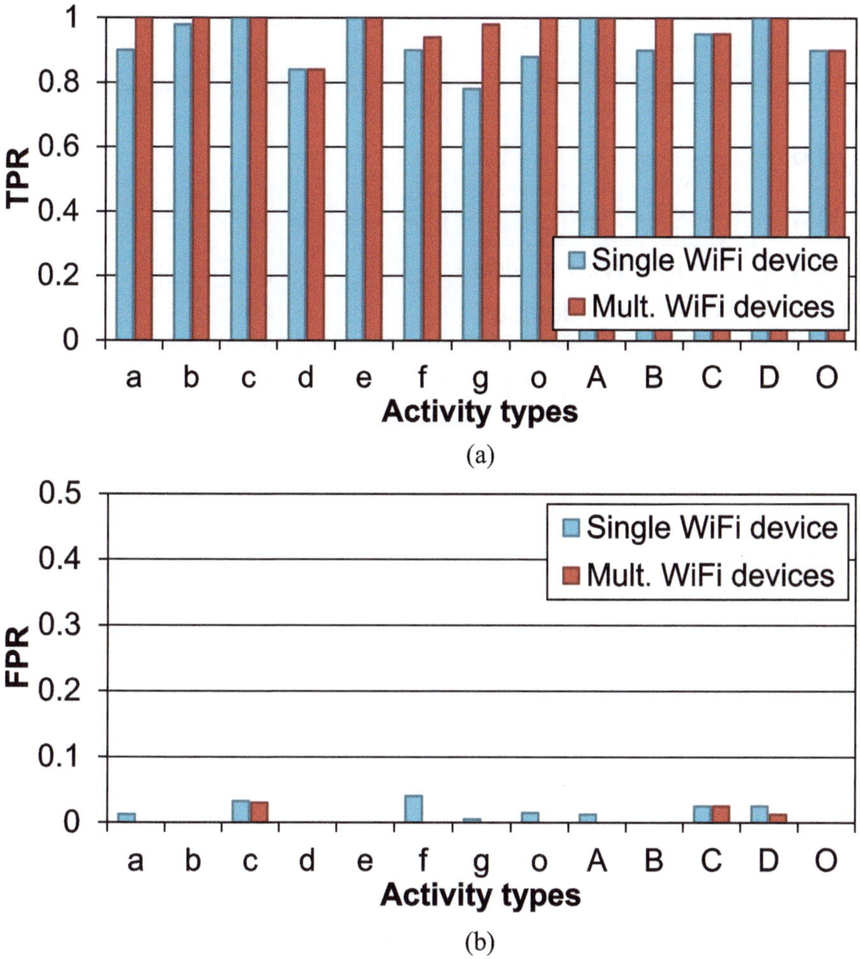

Fig. 2.12 True positive rate and false positive rate, in-place and walking activity recognition in 1-bedroom apartments. (**a**) TPR, 1-bedroom apartment. (**b**) FPR, 1-bedroom apartment

for identifying different activities in two apartments—an average FPR of about 0.6%. The walking activities have higher FPRs which are around 0.8% for both apartments. This is primarily because it is hard to follow exactly the same trajectory every time, and people's body movements maybe different from time to time when walking, such as the sequences of waving arms and alternating two legs. We also observe that the FPRs for identifying all activities are ranging from 0 to 2.5% in both apartments with an average TPR as high as 97% as shown in Figs. 2.12a and 2.13a. The results indicate that our system is robust in identifying both in-place and walking activities in two apartments of different sizes.

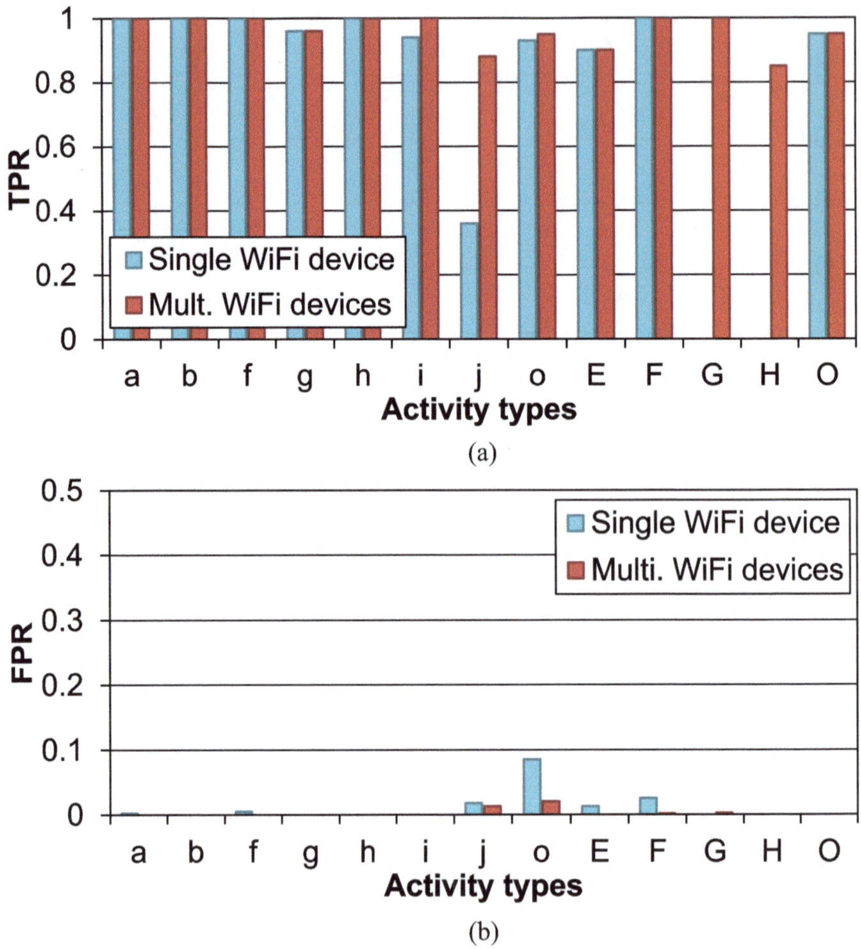

Fig. 2.13 True positive rate and false positive rate, in-place and walking activity recognition in 2-bedroom apartments. (**a**) TPR, 2-bedroom apartment. (**b**) FPR, 2-bedroom apartment

2.6.3.2 Activity Identification with Single WiFi Device

To further show the capability of the system in activity recognition with limited WiFi devices at home, we experiment with only one WiFi device connecting with one single AP. This is a challenging scenario as with only one AP and one WiFi device, the signal affected by the human body may become very weak after going through several walls. We place the WiFi device at one of the previous locations to sense the activities in both apartments. We find that our system is capable of identifying activities accurately when placing a single AP at an appreciate location. In particular, Figs. 2.12a and 2.13a show that the TPRs of identifying both in-place and walking activities are in general over 90% with FPRs less than 5% in the one-bedroom apartment.

In the two-bedroom apartment, most in-place activities have TPRs over 90% and FPRs less than 2%, except the activity *sleeping*. This is because sleeping involves little body movements, thus having less effects on altering multipath environments. In addition, Figs. 2.12b and 2.13b show that the TPRs for walking activities G and H are 0 because they do not generate large moving variances and are classified as *empty room* in the pre-constructed profiles. This is because with the WiFi device and the AP separated by several walls, the conducted activities that are far away from either the WiFi device or the AP will have little effect on altering the multipath environment. Besides G and H, the other two walking activities E and F still have TPRs over 90% with FPRs less than 3%.

2.6.3.3 Distinguishing Activities at the Same Location

Given that some activities take place at the same location but with different human postures or body movements (e.g., sleeping/sitting on the bed), we experiment with such in-place activities to evaluate how well the system can distinguish these activities that occur in the same location. We use different numbers of EMD bins to test the impact on the resolution of identifying activities occurring in the same location. Intuitively, a larger number of EMD bins can provide more detailed distribution information. We add two more activities that occur in the same locations as two of the previously considered activities. We therefore experiment with 4 in-place activities in the one-bedroom apartment: sleeping on the *bed*, sitting on the *bed*, receiving calls nearby the *sink* and washing dishes nearby the *sink*. The system compares the measure in-place activity data against 12 profiles (the 10 from Table 2.3 and the two additional ones). We use the worst TPR (minimum TPR of all activity identification) and the worst FPR (maximum FPR of all activity identification), to evaluate the worst-case performance with different numbers of EMD bins. Figure 2.14a and b show the results of identifying different activities in the same location. We find that the system can achieve high accuracy (over 97%) if the number of EMD bins is greater than 8 when different activities took place at the same locations.

2.6.3.4 Activity Recognition Using Wider-band Signals

Next we study the feasibility of extending the system to work with wider-bandwidth channel of 802.11ac. The bandwidth of a 802.11ac channel is 4 times wider than that of 802.11n. The number of available subcarriers thus increases from 56 in 802.11n to 242 in 802.11ac. Larger numbers of subcarriers provided by 802.11ac therefore have potential to capture in-place activities more accurately and reliably. Since 802.11ac shares the same 5 GHz band with 802.11n, we use multiple 802.11n channels to

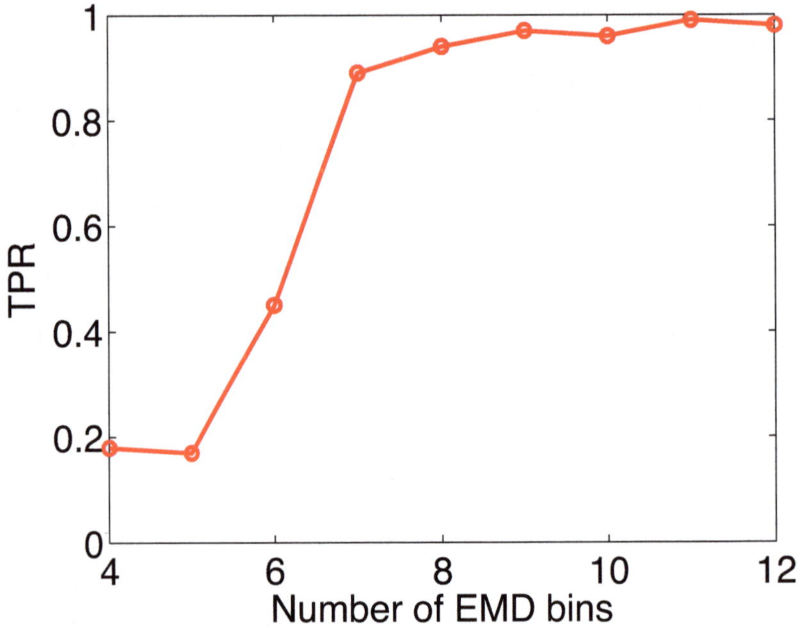

(a)

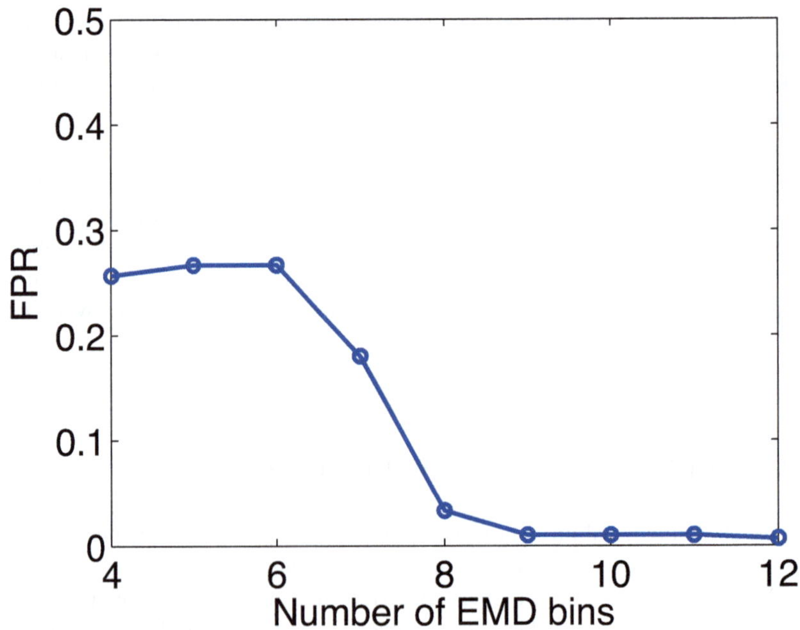

(b)

Fig. 2.14 True positive rate and false positive rate, in worst-case with different numbers of EMD bins

emulate the 802.11ac channel for CSI extraction as no handy tool is available to collect CSI from 802.11ac.

In particular, we use two laptops respectively communicating with two access points to collect CSI measurement from two 802.11n channels (40MHZ) simultaneously at the 5 GHz band. The CSI measurements are off-line synchronized and cascaded in frequency domain to emulate the CSI measurements from a 802.11ac channel (80 MHz). In order to make sure the two 802.11n channels share the same multipath effect, we use two external antennas for the laptops and place them next to each other. The distance between two antennas is about 2 cm, which is smaller than the half wavelength of the 5 GHz WiFi signal (i.e., about 2.8 cm). Similarly, we take the internal antennas of the access points out and bind them together with the distance much less than the half wavelength of the 5 GHz WiFi signal. We experiment with 7 in-place activities in the two-bedroom apartment with the laptops in the living room and the access points in the kitchen as shown in Fig. 2.8.

Figure 2.15 presents the performance comparison of the system with the 802.11n and the emulated 802.11ac channel at 5 GHz band. We find that the system results in higher accuracy under the emulated 802.11ac than 802.11n. This demonstrates the feasibility of improving the recognition accuracy by utilizing wider-bandwidth of 802.11ac. The TPRs for all in-place activities are over 99%. With such high TPRs, the FPRs are still lower than 1% even for two close proximity activities *f: brushing teeth* and *g: taking a bathing*. Furthermore, comparing to the performance of the same setup using 802.11n with one WiFi device, we find that using the 802.11ac channel has about 4% improvement in the worst TPRs (i.e., increases from 94 to 98% for the activity *i: playing video game*). And the worst FPR drops to 0.67% under 802.11ac from 8.5% under 802.11n for *unknown* activities. This indicates that the wider channels (e.g., 802.11ac) can improve the recognition accuracy since it allows measurements over many additional subcarriers.

2.6.3.5 Impact of Traffic Transmission Rate

Since CSI is measured from each of the received packets, the higher packet transmission rate (PTR) results in larger sizes of CSI measurements for characterizing an activity. We thus study the impact of PTR on the system performance. In particular, PTR is changed from 5 pkts/s to 20 pkts/s with a fixed step of 5 pkts/s. As the commercial access points send beacon signals at 10 beacons/s to broadcast their SSID and the connection information, the range of our PTR is thus reasonable and includes the normal transmission rate that is considered to be energy-efficient (10 pkts/s). Figure 2.16 shows the average TPRs and FPRs over all activities with different transmission rates. The increasing and decreasing trends in TPRs and FPRs respectively demonstrate that higher PTR would help to distinguish different activities. We can see that when the PTR is above 10 pkts/s, the average TPRs and FPRs are respectively over 92% and less than 2%, and the improvement of the increased packet rate is less obvious. The results demonstrate that our system is

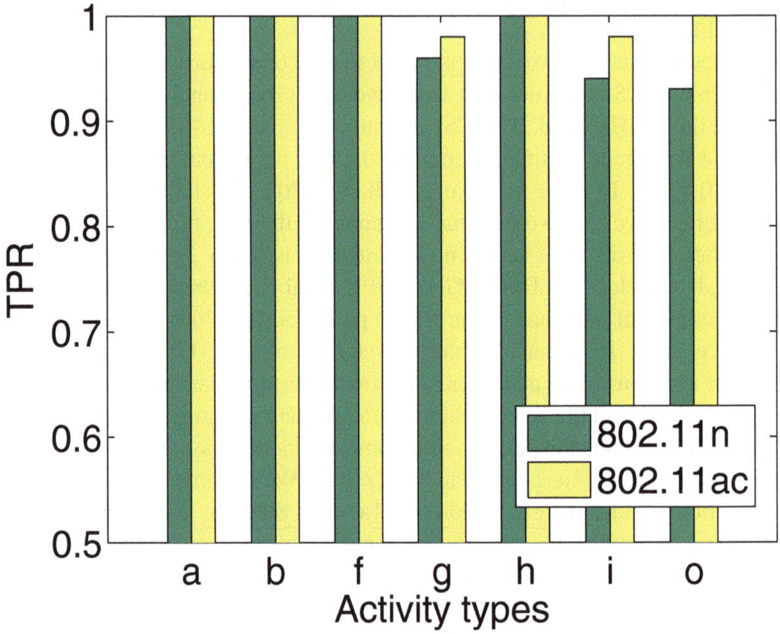

(a)

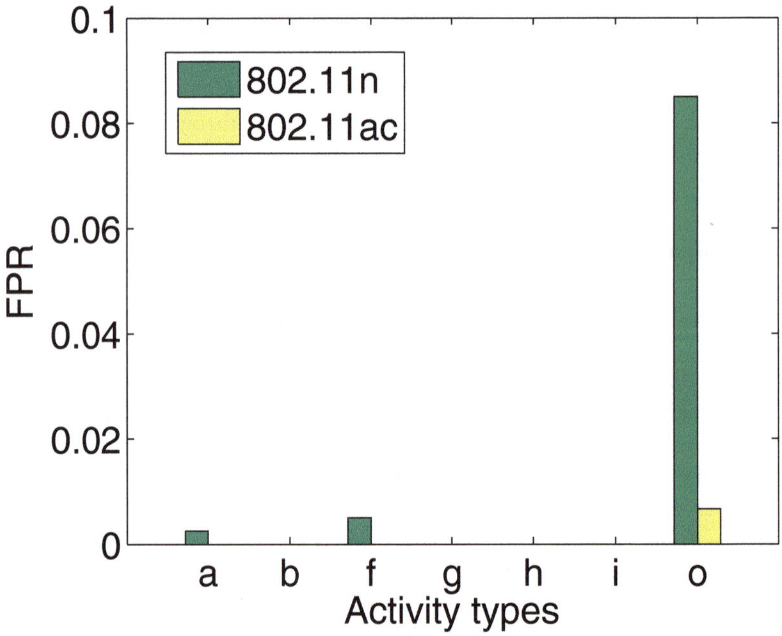

(b)

Fig. 2.15 True positive rate and false positive rate of activity recognition using 802.11n or emulated 802.11ac channel. (**a**) True positive rate. (**b**) False positive rate

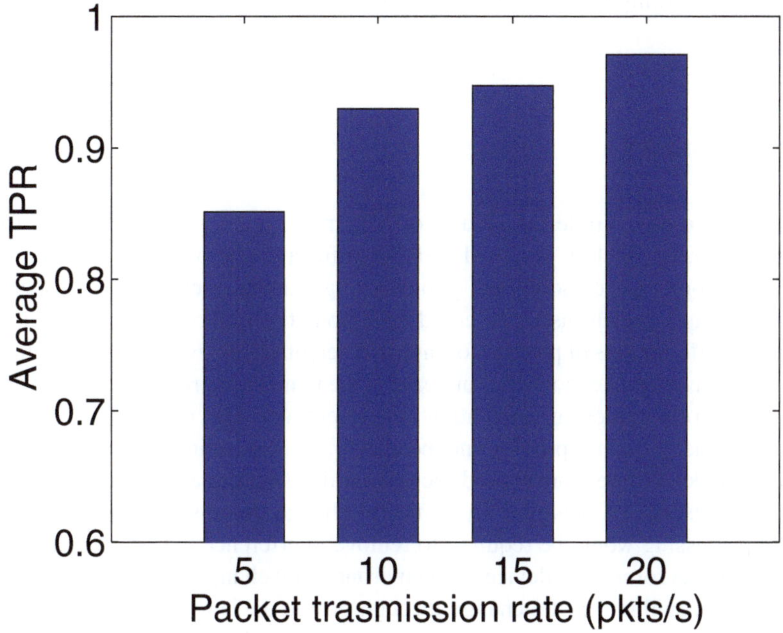

(a)

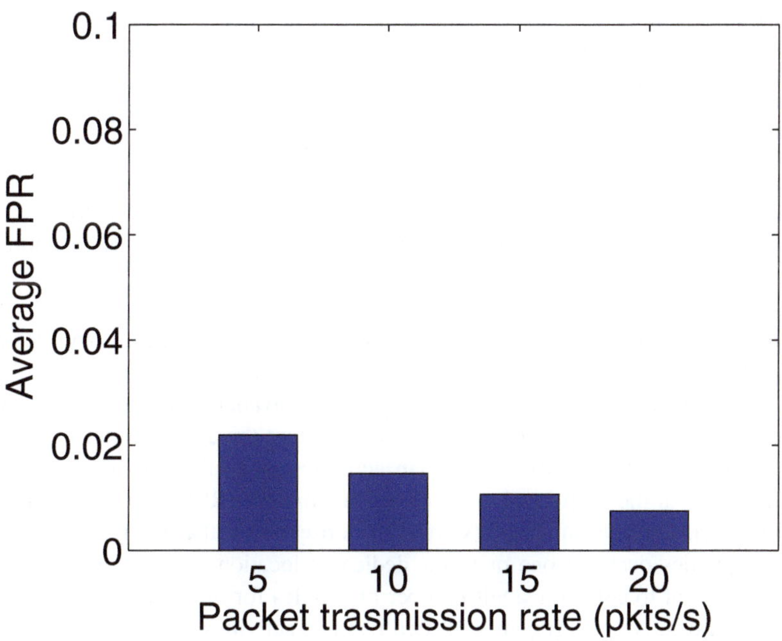

(b)

Fig. 2.16 True positive rate and false positive rate of the system with different PTR. (**a**) Average true positive rate. (**b**) Average false positive rate

capable of working with very low PTR, such as the default beacon packet rate in WiFi.

2.7 Summary

The presence of multiple individuals or pets in the home poses challenges to the current system, which is designed and tested for a single occupant. Detecting the temporary presence of additional people using existing methods and suspending operation during such instances could be a potential improvement. Alternatively, adopting different sets of profiles for multiple persons could be considered, although this would require an exponential increase in the number of profiles needed. Another approach worth exploring is isolating concurrent activities in separate spaces and matching them against profiles independently, by separating effects detected on different links. Future work should focus on addressing these challenges. Additionally, the presence of pets may dynamically change the environment, and further signal processing would be required to remove interference in CSI caused by pets' movement. As for mobile devices and environmental changes, if a device is moved, the system could detect the change through profile deviations or other movement detection techniques and trigger activity profile updates. Smaller environment changes could be handled similarly. The system's constant traffic requirement can be managed by utilizing existing traffic measurements during periods of link usage and creating dummy traffic to invoke device responses when links are not in use. Furthermore, this work has primarily focused on activities linked to specific locations in the home, allowing for a limited set of profiles that combine location and activity information. Exploring the possibility of using profiles to detect the same activity in different locations, as well as distinguishing between different activities in the same location, remains an open question that requires further investigation. Additionally, considering a larger number of activities in the same location and assessing the impact of changes in the propagation environment would contribute to a better understanding of the technique's limitations.

In this chapter, we exploit the prevalence of WiFi infrastructure and design a system to perform device-free location-oriented activity identification by utilizing the fine-grained channel state information (CSI) available in the existing WiFi protocol (i.e., 802.11n). We find that CSI can capture the unique patterns of small-scale fading caused by different human activities at a subcarrier level, which is not available in the traditional received signal strength (RSS) extracted at the per packet level. Our system benefits from the observation that many important in-home activities occur in one or a few dedicated locations and that it is therefore often sufficient to collect a small number of profiles for these activities in each of these locations. An experiment with two pairs of activities that occur in the same location, however, also showed strong potential for the technique to identify a set of activities that occur in the same place. The designed system applies matching algorithms to compare the CSI measurements against known profiles to identify the activity. Extensive experiments in two different-sized apartments demonstrate that the system is effective in distinguishing a number of daily activities, and that it can achieve a detection rate as high as 92% with a single AP and only one WiFi device. In addition, we also show how trends to wider-bandwidth channels (e.g., 802.11ac) will enhance activity recognition performance further.

References

1. Adib, F., Katabi, D.: See through walls with wifi! In: Proceedings of the ACM SIGCOMM 2013 conference on SIGCOMM (2013)
2. Adib, F., Kabelac, Z., Katabi, D., Miller, R.C.: 3d tracking via body radio reflections. In: Proceedings of the 11th USENIX Conference on Networked Systems Design and Implementation (NSDI) (2014)
3. Azizyan, M., Constandache, I., Roy Choudhury, R.: Surroundsense: mobile phone localization via ambience fingerprinting. In: Proceedings of the 15th annual international conference on Mobile computing and networking (ACM MobiCom) (2009)
4. Bahl, P., Padmanabhan, V.N.: Radar: an in-building RF-based user location and tracking system. In: Proceedings of the IEEE International Conference on Computer Communications (IEEE INFOCOM), pp. 775–784 (2000)
5. Banerjee, N., Agarwal, S., Bahl, P., Chandra, R., Wolman, A., Corner, M.D.: Virtual compass: relative positioning to sense mobile social interactions. In: Pervasive (2010)
6. Chang, H.l., Tian, J.b., Lai, T.T., Chu, H.H., Huang, P.: Spinning beacons for precise indoor localization. In: Proceedings of the 6th ACM Conference on Embedded Network Sensor Systems (ACM SenSys) (2008)
7. Gardner, E.S.: Exponential smoothing: the state of the art. J. Forecasting **4**(1), 1–28 (1985)
8. Goswami, A., Ortiz, L.E., Das, S.R.: Wigem: a learning-based approach for indoor localization. In: Proceedings of the Seventh COnference on emerging Networking EXperiments and Technologies (ACM CoNEXT) (2011)
9. Halperin, D., Hu, W., Sheth, A., Wetherall, D.: Tool release: gathering 802.11 n traces with channel state information. ACM SIGCOMM Comput. Commun. Rev. **41**(1), 53–53 (2011)
10. Hong, J., Ohtsuki, T.: Ambient intelligence sensing using array sensor: Device-free radio based approach. In: Proceedings of the 2013 ACM conference on Pervasive and ubiquitous computing adjunct publication (UbiComp '13 Adjunct) (2013)
11. IEEE std. 802.11n-2009: Enhancements for higher throughput (2009). Http://www.ieee802.org
12. Joshi, K., Hong, S., Katti, S.: Pinpoint: localizing interfering radios. In: Proceedings of the 10th USENIX conference on Networked Systems Design and Implementation (NSDI) (2013)
13. Keally, M., Zhou, G., Xing, G., Wu, J., Pyles, A.: Pbn: towards practical activity recognition using smartphone-based body sensor networks. In: Proceedings of the 9th ACM Conference on Embedded Networked Sensor Systems (ACM SenSys), pp. 246–259 (2011)
14. Kleisouris, K., Chen, Y., Yang, J., Martin, R.P.: Empirical evaluation of wireless localization when using multiple antennas. IEEE Trans. Parallel Distrib. Syst. (IEEE TPDS) **21**(11), 1595–1610 (2010)
15. Kosba, A.E., Saeed, A., Youssef, M.: Rasid: a robust wlan device-free passive motion detection system. In: Proceedings of the International Conference on Pervasive Computing and Communications (IEEE PerCom) (2012)
16. Lei, J., Ren, X., Fox, D.: Fine-grained kitchen activity recognition using rgb-d. In: Proceedings of the 2012 ACM Conference on Ubiquitous Computing (ACM UbiComp) (2012)

17. Li, L., Hu, P., Peng, C., Shen, J., Zhao, F.: Epsilon: a visible light based positioning system. In: Proceedings of the 11th USENIX Conference on Networked Systems Design and Implementation (NSDI) (2014)
18. Liu, H., Gan, Y., Yang, J., Sidhom, S., Wang, Y., Chen, Y., Ye, F.: Push the limit of wifi based localization for smartphones. In: Proceedings of the 18th Annual International Conference on Mobile Computing and Networking, pp. 305–316 (2012)
19. Microsoft: X-box kinect (2010). http://www.xbox.com
20. Philips: Philips lifeline (2006). http://www.lifelinesys.com/content/
21. Pu, Q., Gupta, S., Gollakota, S., Patel, S.: Whole-home gesture recognition using wireless signals. In: Proceedings of the 19th Annual International Conference on Mobile Computing & Networking (ACM MobiCom) (2013)
22. Rabiner, L.R., Juang, B.H.: Fundamentals of Speech Recognition, vol. 14. PTR Prentice Hall, Englewood Cliffs (1993)
23. Rousseeuw, P.J., Leroy, A.M.: Robust Regression and Outlier Detection. John Wiley & Sons, New York (2005)
24. Rubner, Y., Tomasi, C.: Perceptual Metrics for Image Database Navigation. Springer Science & Business Media, Berlin (2001)
25. Seifeldin, M., Saeed, A., Kosba, A.E., El-Keyi, A., Youssef, M.: Nuzzer: a large-scale device-free passive localization system for wireless environments. IEEE Trans. Mobile Comput. **12**(7), 1321–1334 (2012)
26. Sen, S., Radunovic, B., Choudhury, R.R., Minka, T.: You are facing the mona lisa: spot localization using phy layer information. In: Proceedings of the 10th International Conference on Mobile Systems, Applications, and Services, pp. 183–196 (2012)
27. Sigg, S., Shi, S., Ji, Y.: Rf-based device-free recognition of simultaneously conducted activities. In: Proceedings of the 2013 ACM Conference on Pervasive and Ubiquitous Computing Adjunct Publication, pp. 531–540 (2013)
28. Technology, A.: Grandcare systems. http://www.grandcare.com/
29. Ten Holt, G.A., Reinders, M.J., Hendriks, E.A.: Multi-dimensional dynamic time warping for gesture recognition. In: Thirteenth Annual Conference of the Advanced School for Computing and Imaging, vol. 300, p. 1 (2007)
30. Van Kasteren, T., Englebienne, G., Kröse, B.J.: An activity monitoring system for elderly care using generative and discriminative models. Pers. Ubiquitous Comput. **14**, 489–498 (2010)
31. Wang, J., Katabi, D.: Dude, where's my card? rfid positioning that works with multipath and non-line of sight. In: Proceedings of the ACM SIGCOMM 2013 conference on SIGCOMM, pp. 51–62 (2013)
32. Wilson, J., Patwari, N.: Radio tomographic imaging with wireless networks. IEEE Trans. Mobile Comput. **9**(5), 621–632 (2010)
33. Xiong, J., Jamieson, K.: Arraytrack: A fine-grained indoor location system. Usenix (2013)
34. Yang, J., Chen, Y.: Indoor localization using improved rss-based lateration methods. In: GLOBECOM 2009–2009 IEEE Global Telecommunications Conference, pp. 1–6. IEEE (2009)
35. Yang, J., Ge, Y., Xiong, H., Chen, Y., Liu, H.: Performing joint learning for passive intrusion detection in pervasive wireless environments. In: 2010 Proceedings IEEE INFOCOM, pp. 1–9. IEEE (2010)
36. Yang, J., Lee, J., Choi, J.: Activity recognition based on rfid object usage for smart mobile devices. J. Comput. Sci. Technol. **26**(2), 239–246 (2011)
37. Yang, S., Dessai, P., Verma, M., Gerla, M.: Freeloc: Calibration-free crowdsourced indoor localization. In: 2013 Proceedings IEEE INFOCOM, pp. 2481–2489. IEEE (2013)
38. Yatani, K., Truong, K.N.: Bodyscope: a wearable acoustic sensor for activity recognition. In: Proceedings of the 2012 ACM Conference on Ubiquitous Computing, pp. 341–350 (2012)
39. Youssef, M., Agrawala, A.: The horus wlan location determination system. In: Proceedings of the 3rd International Conference on Mobile Systems, Applications, and Services, pp. 205–218 (2005)

40. Youssef, M., Mah, M., Agrawala, A.: Challenges: device-free passive localization for wireless environments. In: Proceedings of the 13th Annual ACM International Conference on Mobile Computing and Networking, pp. 222–229 (2007)
41. Zhao, Y., Patwari, N., Phillips, J.M., Venkatasubramanian, S.: Radio tomographic imaging and tracking of stationary and moving people via kernel distance. In: Proceedings of the 12th International Conference on Information Processing in Sensor Networks, pp. 229–240 (2013)

Chapter 3
Personalized Fitness Assistance Using Commodity WiFi

Building upon the insights gained from the exploration of activity monitoring using WiFi signals, this chapter now focuses on the development of personalized fitness assistance using WiFi signals specifically designed for home/office settings. Traditional approaches, which often rely on costly wearable sensors or specialized hardware installations, can be intrusive and uncomfortable for users. In light of these limitations, our research aims to provide a more affordable and user-friendly solution. To achieve this, in this chapter, we develop a personalized device-free fitness assistant system that utilizes existing WiFi infrastructure in home/office environments. Our system aims to provide personalized fitness assistance by differentiating individuals, automatically recording fine-grained workout statistics, and assessing workout dynamics. Using deep learning techniques, we perform individual identification based on workout interpretation, enabling tailored assistance. Our system also analyzes short and long-term workout quality and provides insightful workout reviews for users to enhance their exercises. We ensure system robustness through a spectrogram-based workout detection algorithm and a Cumulative Short Time Energy (CSTE)-based workout segmentation method. To assess the performance of our system, we conducted extensive experiments with a significant number of participants. The results reveal a high level of accuracy in both workout recognition and individual identification, underscoring the effectiveness of our system in providing personalized fitness assistance.

The rest of the chapter is organized as follows. We present the research background in Sect. 3.1 and discuss related work in Sect. 3.2. Next, in Sect. 3.3, we provide the design of the personalized fitness assistant system. In Sect. 3.4, we focus on workout recognition using WiFi. In Sect. 3.5, we delve into the personalized workout interpretation via deep learning. Moving forward, we describe the smart workout assessment using WiFi in Sect. 3.6. In Sect. 3.7, we introduce the system implementation and conduct the evaluation. Finally, we provide a discussion and conclude our work in Sect. 3.8.

X. Guo et al., *Mobile Technologies for Smart Healthcare System Design*,
Wireless Networks, https://doi.org/10.1007/978-3-031-57345-3_3

3.1 Background

Nowadays, people pay more attention to their physical health because the accelerated pace of life and increasing work pressure have compelled many individuals to adapt to a sedentary lifestyle. They either sit all day working on computers or spend long hours with phones. Such sedentary lifestyles often lead to many chronic illnesses (e.g., obesity), which have a significantly negative impact on the quality of people's lives. As a result, people increasingly exercise regularly. However, there are few workout options for the work-at-home people or office workers because they often cannot find enough time to exercise at dedicated places (e.g., the gym). Thus, many people gradually resort to exercising at home/office, which is more convenient without space and time constraints, to exercise and maintain their health. Furthermore, people also like to record their exercise details to keep track of their fitness plans. For example, a user performs various exercises such as free weights with dumbbells, stretches, riding a stationary bike, and running on a treadmill. The corresponding exercise statistics could infer meaningful health-related information (e.g., calories burned). It is common for people to not always stick to their fitness plans due to the lack of guidance from exercise experts in home/office environments. Therefore, in this chapter, we take one step further to develop a smart exercise assistant system that facilitates personal workout monitoring and assessment, targeting the home/office environment.

Traditional solutions on workout assistance rely on hiring personal coaches, which incur high cost, and are mostly not available in home/office environments. There is a new trend of utilizing smartphones and fitness trackers [11] to perform workout monitoring including step counting and multi-sport tracking. These approaches require users to wear smart devices all the time and cannot judge whether the users perform exercise correctly. The details on workout monitoring are critical to help the people correct their exercise postures, and thereby achieve their fitness goals. Incorrect postures may cause unnecessary injury or degrade the efficiency of muscle building. Recently, dedicated hardware and sensors (i.e., inertial sensors, RFID tags [10]) are deployed to track users' exercise records. In particular, FEMO [10] proposes a free-weight exercise monitoring system by attaching passive RFID tags on the dumbbells and leveraging the Doppler shift profile. FitCoach [12] develops a workout recognition and review scheme leveraging the inertial sensors embedded in smartphones or smartwatches. However, it is hard to require people, especially seniors, to wear these devices during exercises, and it is desirable to automatically recognize workout and provide recommendations. Therefore, we seek a solution that is device-free to provide fine-grained personalized fitness assistance. We find that Channel State Information (CSI) [13, 14, 17, 28], embedded in WiFi signals, is a desirable candidate to facilitate workout interpretation and workout recommendation without attaching any devices to users. Because of the prevalence of WiFi infrastructures in home/office environments, it is possible to capture people's activities without their participation. Furthermore, to provide a personalized fitness assistance, it is critical to identify each individual since people may choose a shared environment, either in a family environment or in an office space, to exercise. Therefore, our system should derive salient features that can perform individual identification even at a shared space.

In order to extract unique features from CSI that can identify each individual's movement, we resort to deep learning technique, which have demonstrated their capability in other fields such as image processing [27, 31] and natural language processing [9, 22]. We believe the multi-layer design in deep learning [16, 23] could provide distinctive features for individual identification and workout interpretation. Furthermore, people perform non-workout activities throughout the day such as typing in front of computers and answering phone calls, so it is important that the designed system has the capability to distinguish workout activities from non-workout ones. We intend to differentiate workout activities by searching for repetitive patterns in CSI readings using an autocorrelation-based method. Additionally, CSI is sensitive to various environmental factors (e.g., environmental noise and locations), thus our system should be robust to external interference other than workout activities. In particular, to adapt to small location changes (e.g., people may not always exercise at the same spot even in the same location), the exercise training profiles are collected around a certain range of a profile location and hence make the trained model more robust. Finally, the system aims to assess workout dynamics to boost the workout efficiency and avoid unnecessary injury. We intend to measure workout intensity and strength by defining two new metrics, and thereby provide desirable workout recommendations to users.

To summarize, our system provides two high-level functionalities to enable personalized fitness assistance:

(1) Personalized workout interpretation. We develop a Deep Neural Network (DNN) based model to provide personalized workout interpretation with two tiers of information. Specifically, in the first tier, our system will identify workout types and estimate workout frequencies. Then, the second tier leverages fine-grained latent representatives to further identify individuals. The abstract representation in the deeper layer of a DNN model is beneficial to our system in differentiating individuals because individual identification requires more complex knowledge than workout recognition;

(2) Smart workout assessment. Our system analyzes and assesses a user's workout in terms of its intensity and strength. Specifically, we define two new metrics that depict the short-term and long-term pictures of a user's workout pattern, respectively. *Work-to-Rest-Ratio* measures the complete cycle of a repetition within one set and Repetition-tempo-rate represents the tempo (or speed) at which a user performs a repetition. Then, our system provides workout trends to each user in terms of these two metrics, which the user can correct the exercise form accordingly. This method could also be an accompaniment to just watching and following fitness videos [3] from professionals.

The contributions of this chapter are summarized as follows. We have developed a personalized device-free fitness assistant system for home/office scenarios that utilizes existing WiFi infrastructure without requiring active user participation.

This system is capable of differentiating individuals, enabling personalized fitness assistance with comprehensive workout analysis and smart workout assessment. To address the challenge of multiple individuals sharing the same space, we design a deep learning-based approach that leverages fine-grained latent representations to identify individuals on top of users' workout interpretations. Additionally, we have created a quantitative workout analysis framework that can infer various fine-grained information, such as the workout type, number of sets and repetitions, using a spectrogram-based method for accurate exercise segmentation. Our system goes beyond analysis and offers smart fitness recommendations by automatically assessing exercise postures and providing feedback for posture correction. It can also serve as an early alert system for potential physical health issues. To validate our approach, we deployed a system prototype using a pair of laptops and conducted extensive experiments involving 20 participants over a 10-month period. The results demonstrate the high accuracy of our system in individual identification, exercise recognition, and smart workout assessment.

3.2 Related Work

In general, activity recognition and fitness assistant systems can be broadly categorized as motion sensor-based, vision-based and RF-based. In this part, we review existing studies and compare with our personalized fitness assistant system.

Motion sensors (i.e., accelerometer and gyroscope) embedded in body-attached mobile/wearable devices have been used for both activity recognition [8, 18] and exercise recognition [7, 12]. Specifically, Nuactive [8] and Lasagna [18] recognize human activities through semi-supervised learning and deep neural networks on the captured motion sensor readings, respectively. Additionally, the sensors in customized workout gloves [7] and wearable devices (e.g., smartwatches) [12] are used to recognize exercise types and the number of repetitions. These approaches, however, require users to wear additional devices and are limited to recognize the exercise movements only involving upper body parts such as wrist and arm.

To overcome the aforementioned weaknesses, a couple of studies attempt to recognize human activities with the help of cameras [21, 30]. These approaches either use unsupervised learning or pattern matching on the recorded video frames to achieve fine-grained activity recognition. In addition, video analysis has also been applied to measuring workout dynamics and providing exercise guidance [6, 24]. For instance, Su et al. [24] develop a workout recognition system which assists patients in conducting rehabilitation exercises through profile matching on Kinect readings. Celiktutan et al. [6] develop an exercise recognition and assessment scheme which tracks skeleton geometries with Kinect and quantifies the action goodness. However, these vision-based schemes only work when a user stays within the device's line-of-sight zone and can be significantly affected by the environmental light conditions. In addition, video-based techniques also bring privacy concerns.

Recently, RF-based sensing attracts a considerable attention of many researchers [1, 10, 20] due to the prevalent usage of wireless-enabled devices. WiSee [20] and WiTrack [1] can recognize human gestures and track $3D$ motion of a user using the minute Doppler shift and the round-trip time of flight (ToF) of wireless signals, respectively. Additionally, FEMO [10] recognizes and assesses free-weight workouts by attaching passive RFID tags on the dumbbells and analyzing the Doppler shifts of the received signals. These approaches, however, require dedicated devices (e.g., Universal Software Radio Peripheral (USRP), RFID readers) which limits their applications in practice. Recent studies have shown the potential of using off-the-shelf WiFi to recognize human daily activities [28, 29]. They examine CSI in WiFi signals to capture the environmental changes associated with human activity motions. Although existing WiFi based approaches show intriguing results in identifying general activity types (e.g., walking, standing, sitting), the problem of assessing workout qualities (e.g., strength, speed) and providing exercise feedback remains open. Additionally, comparing with the existing activity-recognition studies (e.g., [28, 29]), which mainly focus on recognizing location-oriented daily activities (e.g., cooking in a kitchen, brushing teeth in a bathroom), this work explores the feasibility of using WiFi to recognize various exercise activities at the same or nearby place and further identify the individual who performs the exercises.

Different from existing work, we design and implement a device-free personalized exercise recognition and assessment scheme leveraging existing WiFi infrastructures. The system provides comprehensive workout interpretation, and differentiates individuals without active user participation. Specifically, we examine channel state information (CSI) embedded in WiFi readings which capture workout dynamics of both free weight and body stretching exercises. Moreover, a workout assessment algorithm is developed to evaluate exercise quality by examining motion speed and strength through frequency domain analysis.

3.3 Personalized Fitness Assistant System Design

3.3.1 Challenges in System Design

In order to design a system that enables personalized fitness assistance using WiFi, a number of challenges regarding how to design mechanisms for comprehensive workout interpretation and smart workout assessment need to be addressed as follows.

Individual Recognition In a shared environment such as a home or office, it's often the case that family members or colleagues take turns participating in workout activities. In these settings, the need for personalized fitness assistance becomes apparent. Our system must have the ability to differentiate between individuals - a task that poses quite a challenge, particularly for a device-free system designed to facilitate personalized fitness assistance. This difficulty arises from the fact that there's no dedicated device affixed to each person to collect the necessary signals related to their distinct movements. For this reason, we are in pursuit of a more universal solution, which can accommodate a group of individuals within such a shared space. It's crucial that our system possesses the capability to distinguish one person from another. By achieving this, we can then tailor our fitness interpretation and assessments to each individual, providing them with a personalized fitness experience.

Fine-grained Workout Interpretation Providing fine-grained workout interpretation using WiFi is also challenging. First, people perform non-workout activities throughout the day. Thus, the designed system should have the capability of distinguishing workout related activities from non-workout ones. Second, in order to provide fine-grained workout interpretation, our system needs to accurately decompose an exercise into pieces of repetitions. Thus, a robust CSI segmentation scheme needs to be integrated into our system. Third, our system also needs to handle a common situation where a user may perform workout at a slightly shifted location (e.g., one foot away) from the location where his training profiles are collected. This is challenging because CSI readings are sensitive to location changes, which could significantly degrade the system performance if careful design consideration is not taken.

Smart Workout Assessment Improper and inconsistent workout activities may hinder muscle development efficiency and potentially result in avoidable injuries. However, creating mechanisms for workout assessments using CSI readings in a device-free design poses a significant hurdle. To address this, we introduce two workout-related metrics. One is applied at the level of individual repetitions, and the other considers the overall exercise to provide a holistic workout assessment. These assessments can provide valuable feedback to users, enabling them to make necessary adjustments to their postures in following exercises. The intention behind these metrics is to ensure that each repetition and every set is conducted correctly and effectively. By doing so, we aim to promote the optimal efficiency of workouts while reducing the risk of injuries. This way, users can fully reap the benefits of their workout activities without compromising their safety.

3.3.2 Overview of the Personalized Fitness Assistance System

In this part, we devise a personalized, device-free fitness assistant system that leverages the existing WiFi infrastructure. The key idea is to utilize fine-grained Channel State Information (CSI), readily accessible from standard WiFi devices, to accurately portray personalized workout statistics and assess workout dynamics. To this end, we first define two specific terms that characterize workout activities: *rep* and *set*. A rep (repetition) refers to a single, full motion cycle of a specific exercise. A set, on the other hand, is a sequence of consecutive repetitions. Usually, a user

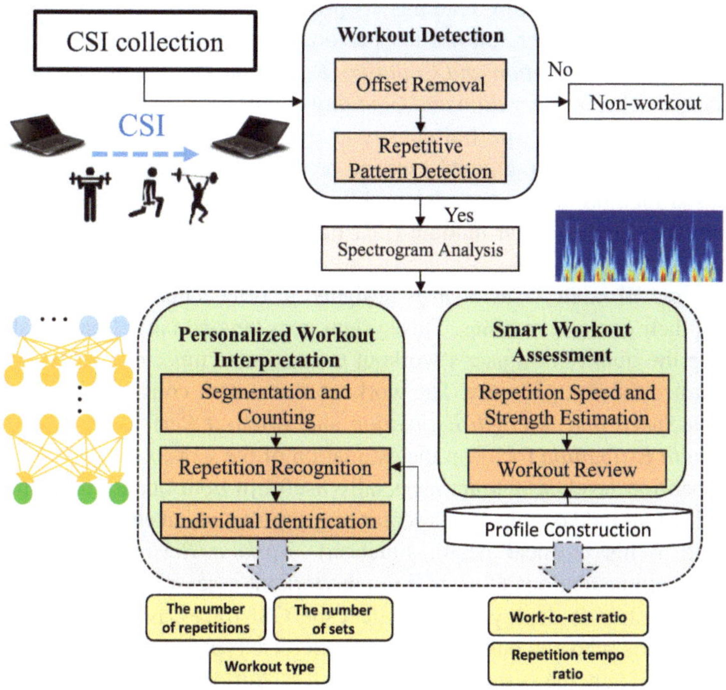

Fig. 3.1 System flow of the designed personalized fitness assistance using commodity WiFi

is advised to perform a workout exercise consisting of several sets to efficiently build muscle and maintain a fit physique. Given these inherent characteristics of a workout, we anticipate that we can observe repetitive CSI patterns because of the repetitive movements from different parts of a body during workouts. Furthermore, minute movements of different workouts have distinct impacts on CSI and thus these unique features of a particular workout can be extracted via CSI analysis.

As illustrated in Fig. 3.1, the designed system takes as input CSI readings which can be directly extracted from WiFi cards [14]. Our system first performs *Workout Detection* to differentiate workout-related activities from non-workout ones based on the discovery of periodical patterns. Specifically, it first applies a sliding window on the CSI time series and then removes the offset (e.g., mean, linear or polynomial trend) of the corresponding CSI data through *Offset Removal*. After that, *Repetitive Pattern Detection* further detects workout activities based on an autocorrelation calculation of the CSI readings. Once the workout-related activities are identified from CSI readings, the system will then perform *Spectrogram Analysis* by converting the CSI time series to frequency-domain. The spectrogram of CSI readings reflects how the workout energy of each frequency component evolves with time.

Next, our system performs *Personalized Workout Interpretation* and *Smart Workout Assessment*. In particular, the *Personalized Workout Interpretation* performs quantitative analysis of CSI readings to produce workout statistics, which can be used to track if a user follows his personal fitness plan correctly. It contains three modules: *Segmentation and Counting*, *Repetition Recognition* and *Individual Identification*. The *Segmentation and Counting* counts the exercise repetitions based on the cumulative power spectral density analysis of CSI spectrogram. *Repetition Recognition* provides fine-grained exercise recognition at the repetition level via a DNN-based method. Then, our system differentiates different individuals through the *Individual Identification* module (i.e., the deeper layer of the designed DNN model).

The *Smart Workout Assessment* is designed to offer valuable feedback to users regarding their exercise routines. This system goes beyond basic fitness statistics in evaluating the quality of a user's workout to maximize muscle-building efficiency and minimize the risk of injury. The workout assessment consists of two modules, *Repetition Speed and Strength Estimation* and *Workout Review*. *Repetition Speed and Strength Estimation* focus on the estimation of the workout speed and strength at the repetition level, which are especially useful in both quality assessment and abnormal workout detection (e.g., a senior may have a sudden change in his workout speed due to his physical health situation). *Workout Review* module provides workout recommendations to users through workout assessment at repetition level. Before our system is deployed, we collect the CSI traces as the training profiles from the experts who can perform different exercise types with standard intensities and strengths. Then, the system compares each repetition of users' exercise profiles against their standard training profiles or experts who visit gym frequently so that it can provide desirable feedback to the users.

3.4 Fine-grained Workout Recognition

3.4.1 Distinguishing Workouts from Non-workout Activities

In environments like homes or offices where people perform various daily activities, CSI readings will inevitably capture both workout and non-workout activities, such as typing at a computer or simply moving around the room. To provide personalized fitness assistance effectively, it is crucial for our system to distinguish between these different types of activities. To recognize the unique CSI features from workout-related activities, we conduct a preliminary experiment in an office setting with a specific individual. This individual's activities were recorded in a sequence. The person first types at a table, then walks to a location to perform five repetitions of standing biceps curls. Following this, he walks back to the same table and continue typing. Figure 3.2 presents the corresponding CSI amplitude for one subcarrier (specifically, the 5th subcarrier), with each activity's timeframe clearly marked. From this experiment, we can observe clear repetitive patterns in the CSI readings during workout activities, which are notably absent during non-workout activities.

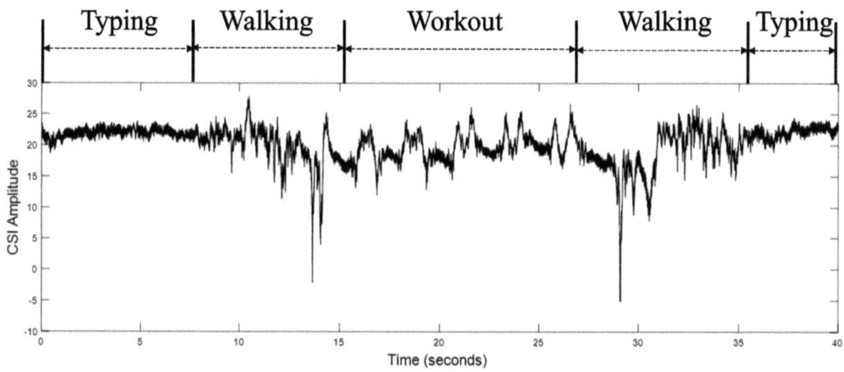

Fig. 3.2 CSI of a series of activities

This distinction illustrates the potential for our system to identify and separate workout activities from other types of movements effectively, an essential step in achieving personalized fitness assistance.

Based on these observations, we design a method to detect workout activities by identifying repetitive patterns in Channel State Information (CSI) readings using the autocorrelation method. Autocorrelation measures the similarity between a signal and itself at a given lag. Therefore, if a repetitive pattern exists, we expect to see a local maximum. Here's how the detection process of repetitive patterns works: Our system first applies a sliding window to the time series of CSI amplitude. For instance, Fig. 3.3a illustrates an 8-second sliding window containing raw CSI readings associated with a workout. We then remove the offset (e.g., mean, linear trend, or polynomial trend) of the raw readings within this window. To do this, we fit a low-order polynomial to the raw CSI data and subtract it, along with the mean value, from the raw CSI readings. Figure 3.3b denotes the data after offset removal. Figure 3.3c shows the results of repetitive pattern detection. Then, a peak (i.e., local maximum) detection algorithm is adopted with an empirical threshold (i.e., 0.2 in this example) to derive the number of repetitions by $N_r = \frac{N_p - 1}{2}$, where N_r is the number of repetitions and N_p is the number of peaks from autocorrelation. Finally, the workout is detected within the specific sliding-window when N_r is larger than a threshold T. Here we assume the workout activities have at least 3 repetitions, thus T is fixed at 3 in our prototype system if not mentioned otherwise.

3.4.2 Recognizing Exercise Repetitions

Once workout activity has been detected, our system aims to recognize each exercise repetition to further generate detailed workout statistics. These statistics, such as the number of sets and repetitions, are integral to understanding the

Fig. 3.3 An example illustrates the process of workout detection. (**a**) Workout raw data. (**b**) Offset removal. (**c**) Repetitive pattern detection

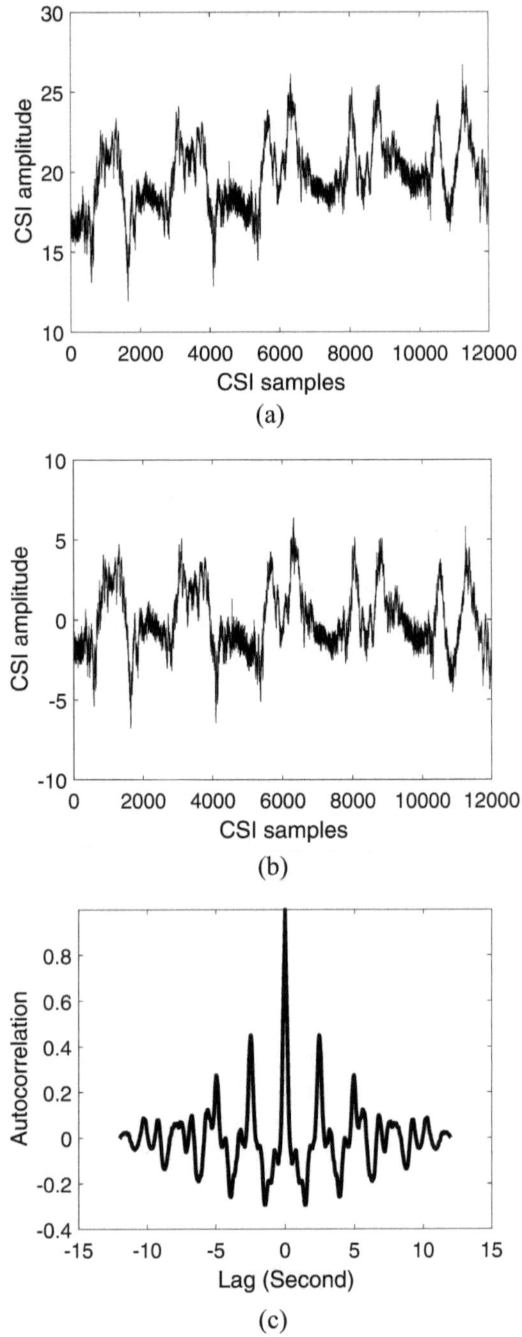

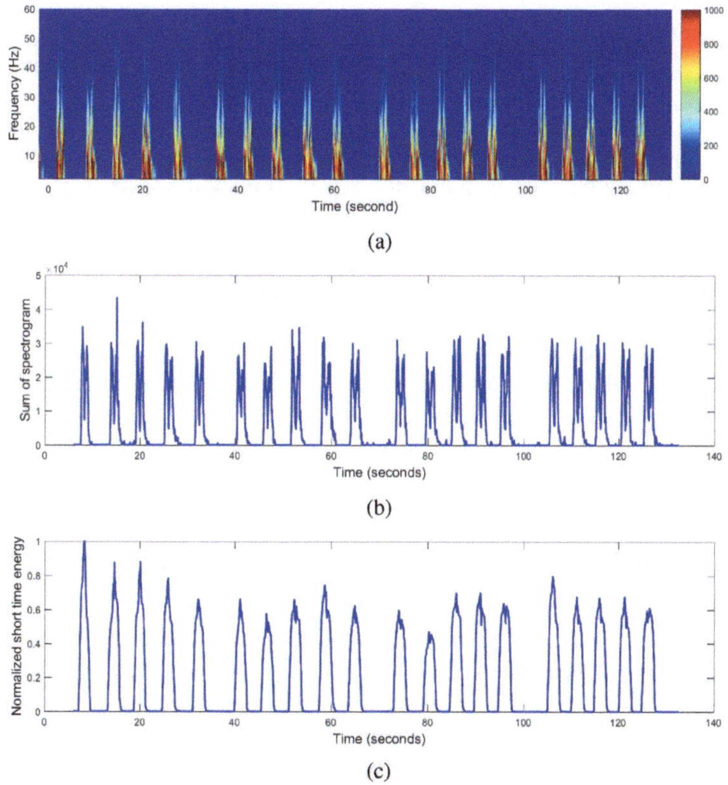

Fig. 3.4 The process of exercise repetition recognition. (**a**) Spectrogram of lateral raise. (**b**) Corresponding Cumulative Power Spectral Density (CPSD). (**c**) The process of exercise repetition recognition

effects of an exercise routine (e.g., calories burned). They are critical in guiding users to design, follow, and adjust their fitness plans. In our design, we opt for spectrogram analysis over time-domain analysis, which is often adversely affected by the presence of interferences, noises, and consistent CSI fluctuations. To verify the effectiveness of spectrogram analysis, we conducted a series of preliminary experiments where volunteers performed four sets of "lateral raises" with five repetitions per set. The corresponding spectrogram in the time-frequency plane reveals a clear repetitive pattern of workout activities as depicted in Fig. 3.4a. We then implement a Cumulative Short Time Energy (CSTE) method to offer detailed workout statistics and further accurately segment each exercise at the repetition level. Specifically, our system first aggregates all power spectral density (PSD) along the frequency dimension in the spectrogram, as demonstrated in Fig. 3.4b. Next, the energy of the cumulative PSD is accumulated again in short sliding window to further make each repetition more distinguishable. Given the accumulated PSD, the normalized short time energy (STE) [4] is derived as:

$$E_{sqr} = \sum_{i=-\infty}^{\infty} [V(i)W(n-i)]^2, \tag{3.1}$$

where $V(i)$ is cumulative PSD, $W(n)$ is the windowing function, and n is the frame shift of samples. Our system identifies all the peaks (i.e., local maximum points) on the normalized STE as shown in Fig. 3.4c, and the number of peaks represents the number of repetitions. Further, we segment each repetition by searching both left and right-hand side of each peak to find zero energy points, and the CSI data between two zero points corresponds to a repetition. We also cluster multiple repetitions into one exercise set if these peaks are far away from others as a user normally takes a longer rest between two consecutive sets. Note that, our system leverages CSI, which provides fine-grained information of wireless channel, and thus it is sensitive to body movement. Therefore, both upper and lower body movement show significant changes in our spectrogram analysis.

3.5 Personalized Workout Analysis Using Deep Learning

In this section, we present a method based on Deep Neural Networks (DNNs) to discern various types of exercises and connect them to their respective users in a common space. The sophisticated patterns generated by DNNs [26], are both stable and resilient to minor alterations in input signals. This attribute suits our system's requirement for a hierarchical setup. Therefore, the designed DNN structure involves two hidden layers, each including an autoencoder and a softmax classifier as show in Fig. 3.5, for workout interpretation and individual identification, respectively. Since each set of workout usually involves multiple repetitions, our system performs repetition-level workout recognition more frequently than set-level individual identification. Furthermore, to reduce computational cost, instead of using the second layer hidden representatives, we leverage the feature abstractions from the first hidden layer to recognize the workout type of each repetition. Specif-

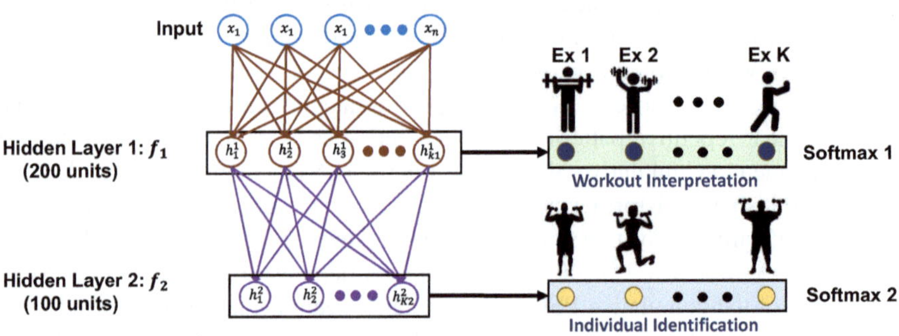

Fig. 3.5 Illustration of the designed DNN architecture

ically, the input vector of DNN consists of features extracted from 30 subcarriers of raw CSI data. At each hidden layer, the autoencoder learns hidden representations from the input vector, and the softmax classifier, which is connected at the end of autuencoder, builds the activity/individual classification model together with the autoencoder with labeled instance. The autoencoders are trained in an unsupervised fashion while the softmax layer is trained with the labeled representations extracted from the autoencoders.

Compared to conventional classifiers like the support vector machine (SVM), our approach using a two-layer DNN can reliably distinguish both workout types and individual identities, notwithstanding the influence of variations in wireless measurements. Typically, Channel State Information (CSI) readings are complicated by the complex shifts in signals caused by slight changes in the propagation path. These shifts are difficult to suppress using a single feature space transformation, such as SVM. Consequently, traditional classifiers like SVM and logistic regression, which require test data to be situated near the hyperplanes learnt from sample profiles, are less effective in reliably identifying individuals and recognizing workouts. To address this, we build a DNN model with multiple hidden layers. This model is capable of capturing robust feature abstractions [25], and reducing the multi-path effect. We further compare our DNN-based method with four other traditional classifiers, including k-nearest neighbors (k-NN), decision tree, random forest and SVM, and discuss the results.

3.5.1 CSI Feature Extraction

To capture the unique characteristics of each type of exercises, it is necessary to extract reliable and efficient features from CSI measurements as the input vector of a DNN model. Since the raw CSI measurements are sensitive to environmental changes, the impact of such ambient interference will be eliminated through obtaining reliable features. In addition, using the features extracted from the raw CSI measurements as input of the DNN model also reduces the computational overhead of our system. There are 8 time domain features extracted from each subcarrier, including *maximum, minimum, mean, kurtosis, skewness, variance, median* and *standard deviation*. Such CSI features are extracted from 30 subcarriers within a single exercise segment, and thus the length of the input vector X is 8×30. In addition, the designed system adopts a high sampling rate of 1000 Hz to ensure the sufficient granularity on capturing human exercise dynamics.

3.5.2 Unveiling Latent Representations with Autoencoders

Given the extracted CSI features, our DNN model first recognizes the exercise type and then identifies individual through analyzing the hierarchical latent representation derived from the input vector. Figure 3.5 illustrates our DNN structure consisting of a two-layer stacked autoencoder [26] with two corresponding softmax classifiers. To determine the number of neurons in each hidden layer, our system iterates through various number of neural units and selects the number that provides the highest cross validation accuracy. The designed DNN structure takes CSI features set X as the input vector and encodes features into hierarchical latent representations (i.e., $y_i (i = 1, 2)$) through activation functions f_i (i=1, 2), where the function outputs can be utilized for workout/identity classification.

The neural units in each DNN layer learn a set of latent representations from the CSI feature inputs in an unsupervised fashion. Specifically, the two hidden layers have 200 and 100 neural units, respectively, and force the network to learn a compressed and sparse representation of the inputs through setting the number of hidden units fewer than the number of inputs n.

The hidden units in each autoencoder map the input vector X into a set of latent representations Y through the following equation:

$$Y = \sigma(wX + b), \tag{3.2}$$

where $\sigma(\cdot)$ is a logistic sigmoid function formulated as $\sigma(z) = \frac{1}{1+e^{-z}}$, and w and b characterize the weight and bias of the autoencoder, respectively. The autoencoders are trained by minimizing the reconstruction errors between X and Y. Particularly, to train an autoencoder, we initialize weights and bias with random numbers. Then, the optimization function Γ in the autoencoder training is defined as follows:

$$\Gamma(X, X') = \frac{1}{K}\sum_{k=1}^{K}(X_k - X_k{}')^2 + \lambda \times \Omega_{weights} + \beta \times \Omega_{sparsity}, \tag{3.3}$$

where K is the number of training samples and X' represents the reconstructed sample from Y using a decoder function. We use $\Omega_{weights}$ and $\Omega_{sparsity}$ to denote the parameters of L_2 regularizer and sparse regularizer [19], which prevent low output values of the neural units. And λ and β are the coefficients of L_2 regularizer and sparse regularizer. Specifically, we denote $\lambda = 0.002$ and $\beta = 4$ for controlling mean squared error for the optimization function Γ. In order to limit the training time while preserving low reconstruction errors for the units in hidden layers, we train the DNN model leveraging a learning rate of 10% and 300 epochs in an unsupervised manner.

3.5.3 Personalized Identification and Workout Analysis

Recognizing individual identities amidst exercise interpretation poses a considerable challenge given the similarities in the gestures people employ across a single type of exercise. Nevertheless, we have discovered that various individuals execute non-identical micro-gestures, which can be detected and differentiated using Channel State Information (CSI). Figure 3.6 presents the CSI measurements for two users partaking in two different exercises. Small variations can be observed in the CSI measurements of two users conducting the same exercise, attributable to the unique characteristics of each user, such as body shape and distinctive behaviors, which uniquely influence the CSI measurements. Thus, we can rely on CSI feature representations to identify each individual. Specifically, we construct the two-layer DNN model by stacking one autoencoder layer on the top of another. Each autoencoder layer outputs latent representations which are abstractions of the input CSI features. Given the feature representations from the two layers, we use two SoftMax [5] functions to perform individual identification and workout Interpretation. The first SoftMax function takes the layer 1 hidden representations as input and recognizes exercise type, while the second SoftMax layer is attached to the second autoencoder and identifies the individual identity. The SoftMax functions are defined as follows:

$$P(C_n|Y) = \frac{P(Y|C_n)P(C_n)}{\sum_{j=1}^{n} P(Y|C_j)P(C_j)}, \tag{3.4}$$

where $P(C_n|Y)$ represents the conditional probability of user identity label C_n given a hidden latent representations Y, and we denote the prior of the same label as $P(C_n)$. $P(Y|C_n)$ indicates the likelihood of the representations Y given class C_n. The values of $P(C_n|Y)$ are constrained by $\sum_{n=1}^{N} P(C_n|Y) = 1$. Each SoftMax function outputs the probability distribution over N profiled users/exercises. Each SoftMax layer is trained through minimizing a mean squared error function, which is defined as:

$$E = \frac{1}{n}\sum_{j=1}^{n}\sum_{i=1}^{k}(t_{ij} - y_{ij})^2, \tag{3.5}$$

where n is the number of observations, and k is the number of users. t_{ji} is the element of a ground truth matrix for training samples and y_{ij} is the hidden representations for the jth observation. Then, we use an optimized function $n = argmax_{n \in N} P(C_n|Y)$ to find a predicted class for the latent representations Y. The training process of Softmax layer runs 400 epochs with the learning rate fixed at 0.15 in a supervised manner to control the training time while preserving classification accuracy.

3.6 Repetition-level Smart Workout Assessment Design

Correct exercise postures will not only reduce the possibility of injury, but also increase the efficiency of muscle building. In addition, any incorrect exercise form may cause some physical health-related problems, especially for the elderly. In this

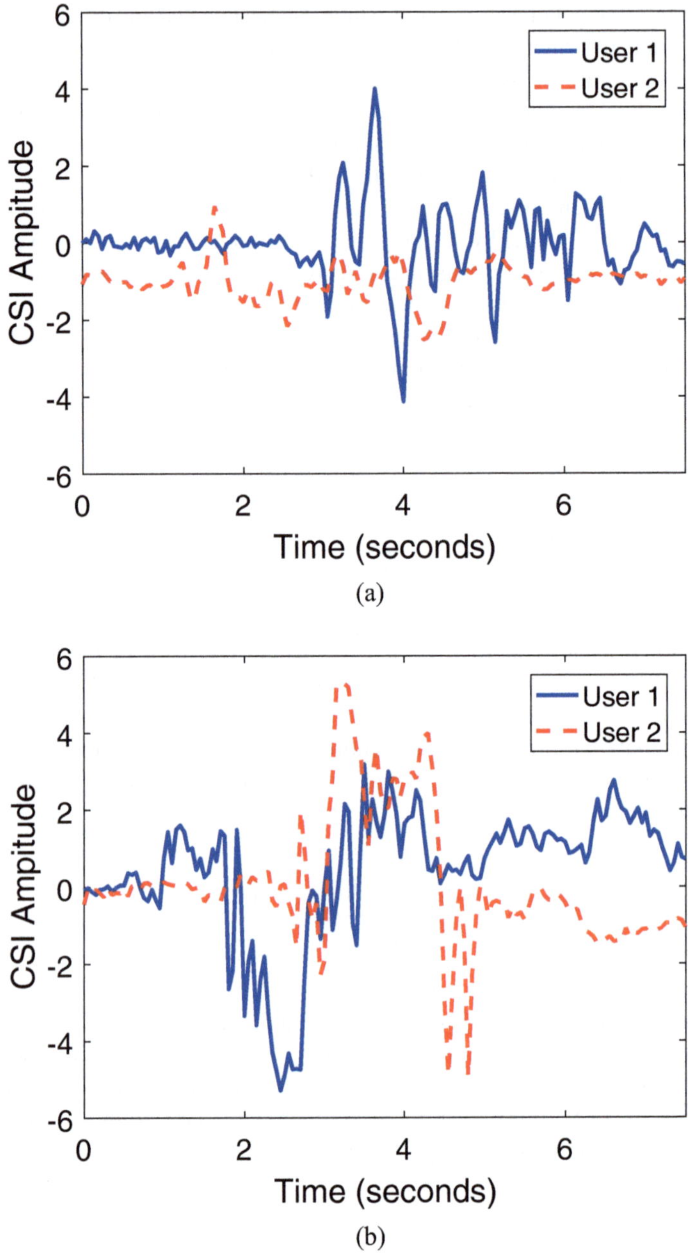

Fig. 3.6 CSI amplitudes of two users performing two types of exercises. (**a**) Spectrogram of lateral raise. (**b**) The process of exercise repetition recognition

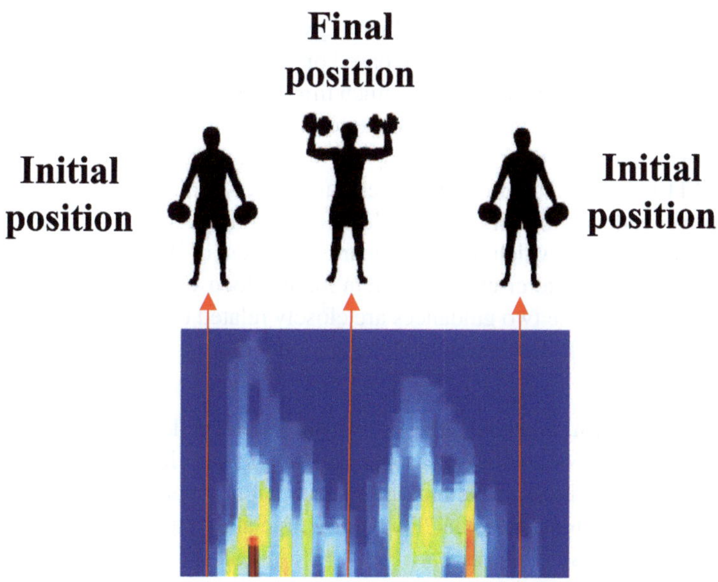

Fig. 3.7 Spectrogram of one repetition

section, we will discuss smart workout assessment based on the analysis at repetition level to help users retain correct exercise postures and thereby achieve their fitness goals.

The Anatomy of a Repetition To perform workout assessment, we first need to have an in-depth understanding of a workout repetition. Basically, a repetition normally consists of a series of body movements from an *initial position* to a *final position* and then back to the *initial position* as shown in Fig. 3.7. The figure shows the spectrogram of a repetition with corresponding movements. In our example, the movement contains *concentric contractions* (i.e., cause muscles to shorten, thereby generating force) and *eccentric contractions* (i.e., cause muscles to elongate in response to a greater opposing force). Good exercise repetitions need to keep a constant rhythm (i.e., the time ratio between concentric contractions and eccentric contractions in our example).

Workout Review and Recommendation In order to achieve effective exercise and avoid injury, it is crucial to customize personal fitness plans by fitness professionals. Such fitness plans often try to regulate the exercise by following the Frequency, Intensity, Time, and Type (FITT) [2] principle of training, which is a set of guidelines that instruct users to set up exercise routines fitting their goals and fitness levels, while maximizing the effects of exercises. Specifically, *Frequency* refers to the frequency of exercise undertaken; *Intensity* refers to the intensity of exercise undertaken; *Time* refers to the time a user spends exercising; *Type* refers to the type of exercise undertaken.

Traditionally, a fitness coach or trainer at gym can keep watching each exercise repetition of a user, and provide advice based on the FITT principle. However, many people who work full time do not have much time to exercise at dedicated place (i.e., the gym). Instead, they often choose to exercise at home or at the office. The *smart workout assessment* module fills the gap between users' needs and fitness plans to meet the FITT principle by providing fine-grained, personalized fitness information, and intuitive feedback to users. The module will automatically provide assessments and recommendations, which relies on the measurement of WiFi CSI readings while users are performing exercises. Our system mainly focuses on perceiving *Intensity* and *Time*, because these two guidances are closely related to exercises in repetition-level. Based on the FITT principle and the anatomy of a rep, we define two metrics as follows.

Work-to-Rest Ratio Workout time in repetition-level reflects how much time is spent on a repetition of a set. It measures the complete cycle of a repetition within one set. To gain efficient muscle building, a user should maintain a consistent ratio between the time of repetitions and the resting time afterwards. Thus, we define the work-to-rest ration as:

$$R_{w2r} = \frac{T_w^{(i)}}{T_r^{(i)}},$$

where $T_w^{(i)}$ is the time duration for the ith workout and $T_r^{(i)}$ is the time duration of the rest followed by the ith workout.

Repetition Tempo Ratio (RTR) Workout intensity usually indicates how much energy is consumed, which can be reflected by a relative percentage of a user's maximum endurance. Specifically, we define the intensity as a ratio between the energy from an initial position to a final position. According to the analysis of the anatomy of a repetition, we found that this ratio can be measured through measuring the time duration from an initial position to a final position, and the time duration of from the final position back to the initial position in a repetition. Thus, we define the repetition tempo ratio as follows:

$$R_{RTR} = \frac{T_{i2f}^i}{T_{f2i}^i},$$

where T_{i2f}^i is the time duration from an initial position to a final position of the ith repetition and T_{f2i}^i is the time duration from the final position back to the initial position of the ith repetition.

Workout Posture Recommendations Based on the assessment results, our system next will provide reasonable workout posture recommendations to help the user to correct exercise gestures. The basic idea is to compare the exercise assessment results of normal users with the ones obtained from expert users in term of the new metrics.

Specifically, our system not only provides the trend of these two metrics across all repetitions, but also shows the upper and lower bounds of the metrics obtained from expert users. Then a user can have a visualized view of his workout assessment and check whether repetition is correctly performed or not. Figure 3.8 plots the workout assessment for a user after he finishes 12 repetitions of lateral raise. The user can observe how each of his repetitions is performed based on work-to-rest ratio and can find the 7th, 8th, 9th repetitions are over the upper bound as shown in Fig. 3.8a. Figure 3.8b provides a different view of each repetition by examining the repetition tempo ratio. The user will find the 5th repetition is over the upper bound and the 10th repetition is below the lower bound. Based on the visualized feedback, the user can adjust his subsequent repetitions by paying attention to those repetitions that are poorly done. In particular, for those repetitions beyond the upper bound of a standard workout, the user needs to extend the rest time after the repetitions, while for those over the upper bound of repetition tempo ratio, the user can increase the intensity from the initial position to the final position.

3.7 System Implementation and Evaluation

3.7.1 Experimental Methodology

Experiment Setup To evaluate the performance of our system, we have developed a prototype using a pair of Dell E6430 laptops, each outfitted with an Intel 5300 802.11*n* WiFi Network Interface Card (NIC). These laptops act as WiFi transceivers. Specifically, both the transmitter and receiver are configured to operate under $Monitor$ mode with a fixed packet rate of 1000 packets/second at a frequency band of 5 GHz. It is important to note that each CSI measurement of the captured packet consists of 30 subcarriers, represented in the form of a complex value. This setup allows us to adequately test the robustness and efficiency of our proposed system.

Data Collection We carried out our experiments with the assistance of 20 volunteers. All of these individuals were college students aged between 22 and 35, among whom 18 are male and 2 are female. We collected their exercise training profiles at multiple points, each located within a foot's distance from a predetermined profile location. The volunteers' workout activities were monitored and analyzed in three distinct indoor locations. Notably, the dimensions of these locations were 6×4 m, 8.3×6.6 m, and 7.3×3.6 m respectively, reflecting common room sizes such as a living room, a spacious family room, and a typical office space. To validate the robustness of our system, our volunteers were asked to perform 10 popular indoor exercises, encompassing free-weight workouts, body stretches, and aerobic exercises. Each volunteer was requested to perform 20 sets of each type of

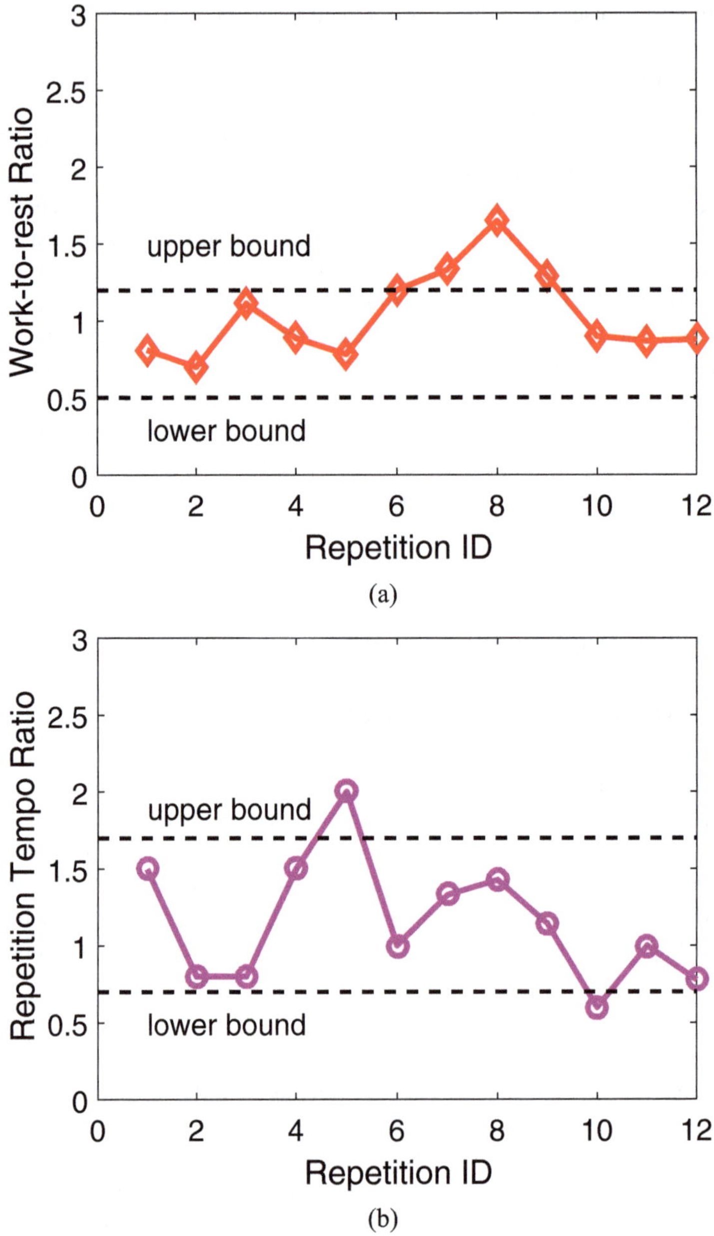

Fig. 3.8 Workout assessment for each repetition based on two metrics. (**a**) Work-to-rest ratio. (**b**) Repetition tempo ratio

exercise per week, with every set comprising of 15 repetitions. This rigorous testing environment was designed to evaluate the performance of our system in real-world conditions thoroughly.

In total, we collect 3013 segments of CSI measurements that are associated with workout activities from the volunteers. For each round of data collection, we ask volunteers to stay in the room for 20 min. During this period of time, a volunteer mimics the scenarios of work-at-home or in the office. Specifically, each volunteer is required to perform workout-related activities for 10 min and any other activities (e.g., with or without repetitive pattern) for the rest of the time. Therefore, the collected CSI readings could include both regular daily activities (e.g., sitting on a chair at work, typing and walking around) and exercise activities from the volunteer. The time duration ratio of the regular daily activities and exercise activities is around $1 : 1$. The design of such a data collection process is to demonstrate that our fitness assistant system has the capability of distinguishing workout-related activities from daily activities.

Evaluation Metrics To quantify the performance of our system, we define four metrics as follows.

Precision Precision is a metric used to gauge the performance of our system in terms of its positive predictive value. Specifically, for a given workout type w, precision is defined as the fraction of sets correctly recognized as workout w (true positives) out of the total number of sets predicted as workout w (true positives plus false positives). In mathematical it is defined as:

$$precision_w = \frac{N_w^T}{N_w^T + M_w^F},$$

where N_w^T represents the number of instances accurately identified as workout w, and M_w^F denotes the number of sets incorrectly identified as workout w that correspond to different workouts in reality.

Recall Recall, also known as sensitivity or true positive rate, is another performance measure that represents the ability of the system to correctly identify positive cases. For a workout w, recall is defined as the proportion of sets correctly identified as workout w (true positives) out of all sets that are actually of workout w (all actual positives). This is calculated as:

$$Recall_w = \frac{N_w^T}{N_w}.$$

F1-Score The F1-score is a metric that provides a singular measure for the accuracy of a system by combining both precision and recall values. It is the harmonic mean of precision and recall, and its value ranges between 0 and 1. A value of 1 implies perfect classification accuracy. In our multi-class scenario, the F1-score for a particular workout w can be computed using the formula:

$$F_1^{(w)} = 2 \times \frac{precision_w \times recall_w}{precision_w + recall_w}.$$

Confusion Matrix The confusion matrix is a tabular representation that shows the classification results of the system. The columns of the confusion matrix represent the actual class (workout type or identity), while the rows represent the predicted class by our system. Each cell in the matrix represents the percentage of sets correctly classified for each exercise type or identity. This matrix is particularly useful in understanding the performance of the classification system, as it provides a clear picture of both the correct predictions and the types of errors made.

3.7.2 Personalized Workout Analysis and Individual Recognition

Workout Interpretation We first examine the performance of workout interpretation based on our DNN model. Figure 3.9a shows the confusion matrix of 10 different workout exercises performed by all volunteers at three different environments. We observe that the average recognition accuracy is around 93% and the standard deviation is 2.6%. Particularly, we find the 8th workout (i.e., pile squat) has a slightly lower accuracy than other types of workout. This is because pile squat involves whole body movement which makes the CSI stream vary a lot from time to time. But our system can still maintain over 89% accuracy. In addition, as shown in Fig. 3.9b, we find that the corresponding precision, recall and F_1 score are all around 93%. The results show that our DNN-based model can achieve high accuracy in workout recognition and thereby confirm the robustness of our system under different environments. Moreover, we investigate workout interpretation performance of a two-layer neural network, which has the same architecture as the two-layer model but leverages the hidden representatives extracted from the second-layer for workout recognition. As shown in Fig. 3.10, we find that the average recognition accuracy is around 91.1% and the standard deviation is 4.6%. Such recognition accuracy is lower than that of our DNN model, because a two-layer model is over-complicated for our workout recognition task. It demonstrates that our system can recognize exercise types with sufficient high accuracy and low computational complexity leveraging hidden representatives derived from the first layer of the DNN model.

Individual Identification Next, we perform individual identification by using our DNN model. In Fig. 3.11, the confusion matrix presents the overall accuracy of individual identification. We find that our system always achieves high identification accuracy across all the volunteers. Particularly, the accuracies for all the individuals are over 92% and the standard deviation is 3.34%. This result validates that

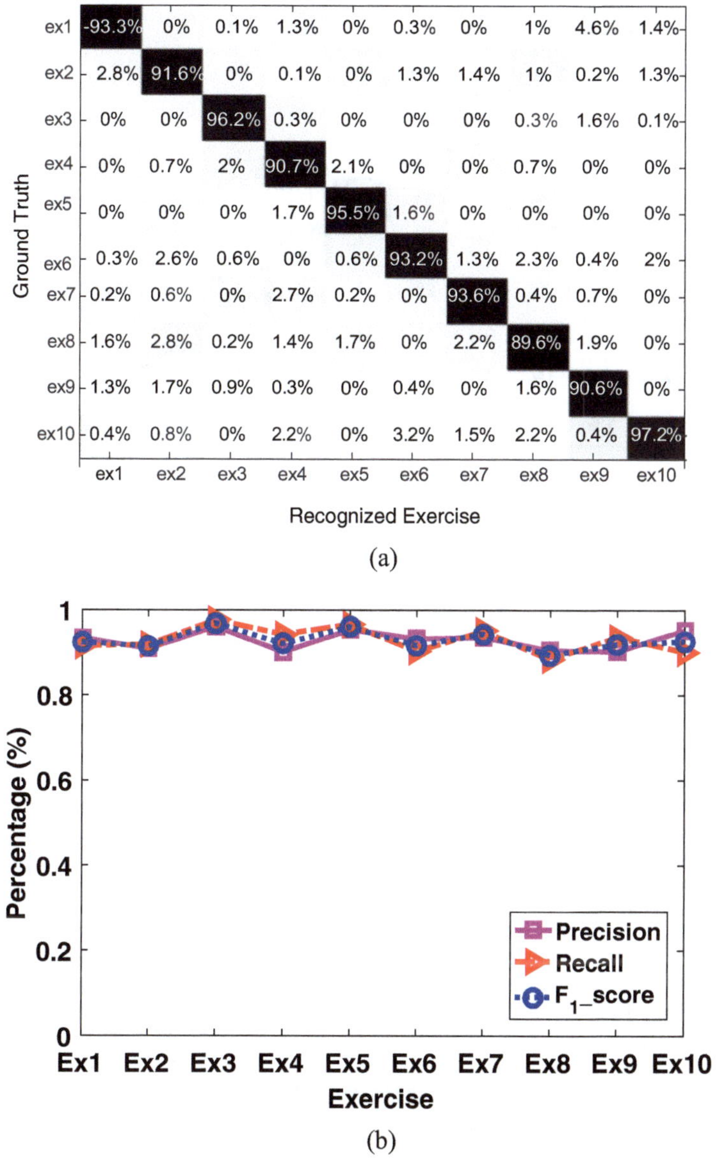

Fig. 3.9 Accuracy of exercise recognition with the DNN model. (**a**) Exercise recognition accuracy. (**b**) Precision/recall/F1-score

our system can identify individuals with high accuracy and therefore, supports personalized fitness assistance. Although the DNN model is sufficiently distinctive in a relative large user population (i.e., 20 people in our current experiments), it

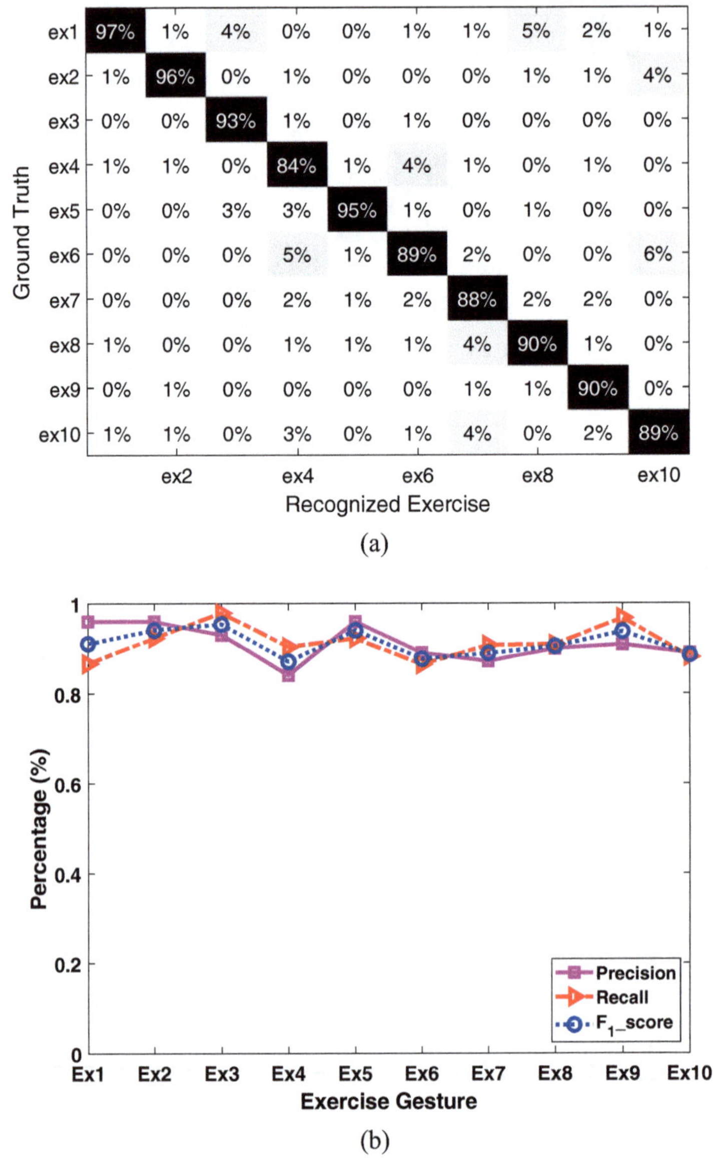

Fig. 3.10 Accuracy of exercise recognition with a separate two-layer DNN model. (**a**) Exercise recognition accuracy (**b**) Precision/recall/F1-score

is not yet clear what the maximum number of users that can be identified by our system. However, our results of 20 people are promising, and this user population size is sufficient for most of the use cases in home or office environments.

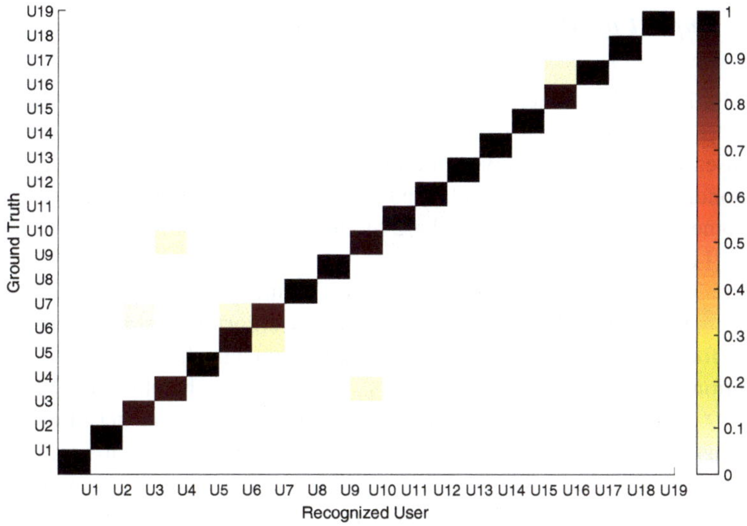

Fig. 3.11 Individual identification accuracy

3.7.3 Personalized Smart Workout Assessment

Our system offers smart workout assessments by comparing each user's exercise patterns with those of expert users, according to the two metrics. Based on this comparison, we generate personalized recommendations for each user. The benchmarks used for comparison are the upper and lower bounds of the two metrics, which are calculated from the performance of the expert users. For this project, we engaged 20 volunteers who each received a workout assessment and made adjustments to their exercise techniques according to the feedback provided by our system. In a more specific experiment, we engaged 6 expert users—individuals who regularly attend the gym and have prior training experience—to perform three sets of exercises with ten repetitions per set for each workout type. We then established the upper and lower bounds for each specific metric, setting the upper bound as the highest value attained by any of the six expert users, and the lower bound as the lowest value. This personalized feedback system received positive reviews from all participants, validating its effectiveness. The volunteers confirmed that our system can accurately analyze workout forms, provide useful feedback, and help them make necessary adjustments for improvement. Through this system, users can optimize their workouts, correct their form, and minimize the risk of injuries. Additionally, the system promotes a greater understanding of the individual user's workout dynamics, contributing to a more effective and satisfying exercise experience.

3.7.4 Impact of Monitoring Device Placements

We study the workout interpretation and people identification scheme by placing the wireless transmitter and receiver at different heights. Specifically, we examine three cases where the transceivers are placed at equal heights, 0.2, 0.8 and 1.3 m, corresponding to the floor, the table, and the top of a cabinet. Furthermore, we also study some real-world scenarios, where the heights of transmitter and receiver are unequal (i.e., 1.3–0.2 m and 0.2–1.3 m).

Figure 3.12a shows the workout recognition accuracy for five different exercises. We observe that our DNN workout recognition algorithm achieves comparable high performances with various transceiver placements. In general, the average recognition accuracies for the five pairs of transceiver heights are 94.7, 99.7, 97.3, 99.6, 98.9%. Specifically, we find that the recognition performances for three transceiver heights (i.e., 1.3–0.2 m, 0.8–0.8 m, and 0.2–0.2 m) achieve over 94% for all five exercises. In addition, we observe that when the transceivers are placed at the height 1.3–1.3 m, exercise 1 and 2 have relatively lower recognition accuracy compared with most of the other transceiver heights. This is because both exercise 1 and 2 involve a gesture of raising the dumbbells to the height of the transmitter (i.e., 1.3 m), resulting in similar multipath and line-of-sight effects. Thus, the CSI readings of these two exercises are very similar and thus the recognition performances are slightly degraded. Beside workout recognition, we also present the individual identification accuracy in Fig. 3.12b. It is encouraging that the identification accuracies for the five cases with equal transceiver heights are all over 97%. The results confirm the designed DNN model is robust to different transceiver heights on workout recognition and people identification.

3.7.5 Impact of Monitoring Device Distances

Furthermore, we also study the workout recognition performance under various transceiver distances, which correspond to different room sizes. We show both the exercise recognition and people identification accuracy of five different exercises in Fig. 3.13. As shown in Fig. 3.13a, our algorithms can achieve good performance for most of the exercises with different transceiver distances. Specifically, the average recognition accuracy for the four distances are: 97.8, 98.9, 96.6, 95.0%. In particular, for the case of the distance 2, 3, and 5 m, the recognition accuracies for the five exercises are all over 94%. For the transceiver distance of $7m$, some exercises (i.e., Ex1 and Ex4) have relative lower recognition accuracy due to the weak signal strength at such a distance. Figure 3.13b shows the people identification accuracy for the four cases of different transceiver distances. We can find that the identification accuracies are all over 99% which validate the reliability of our people identification algorithm at different distances between transmitter and receiver.

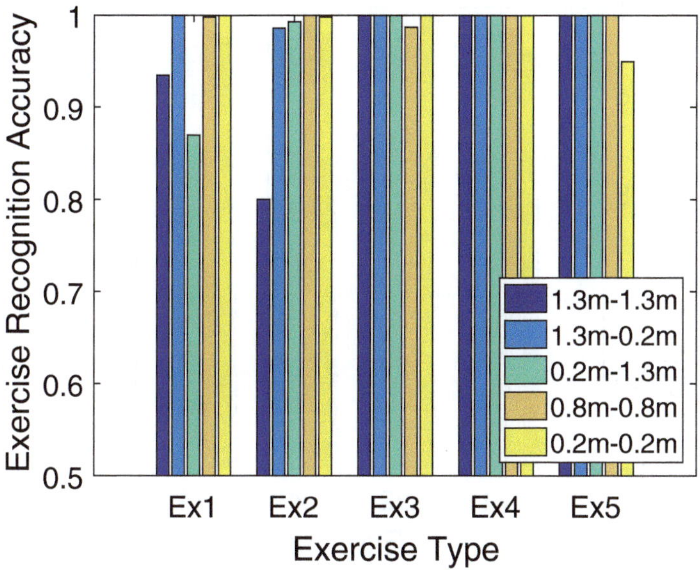

(a)

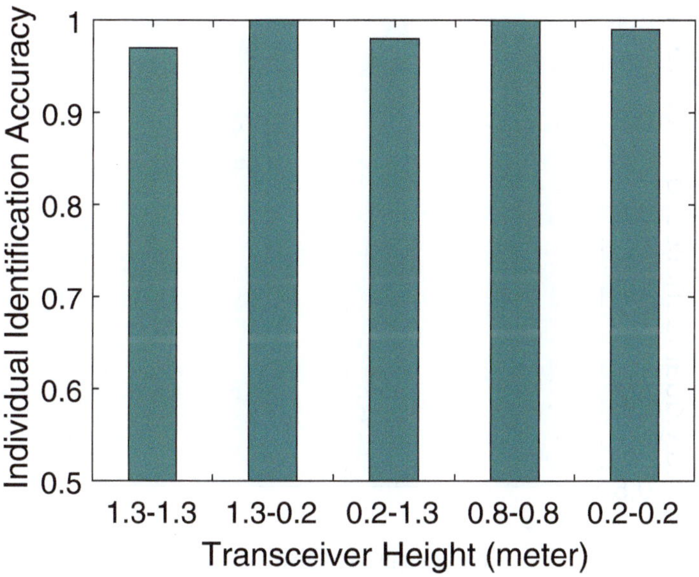

(b)

Fig. 3.12 Impact of transceiver height on exercise recognition and individual identification. (**a**) Workout recognition. (**b**) Individual identification

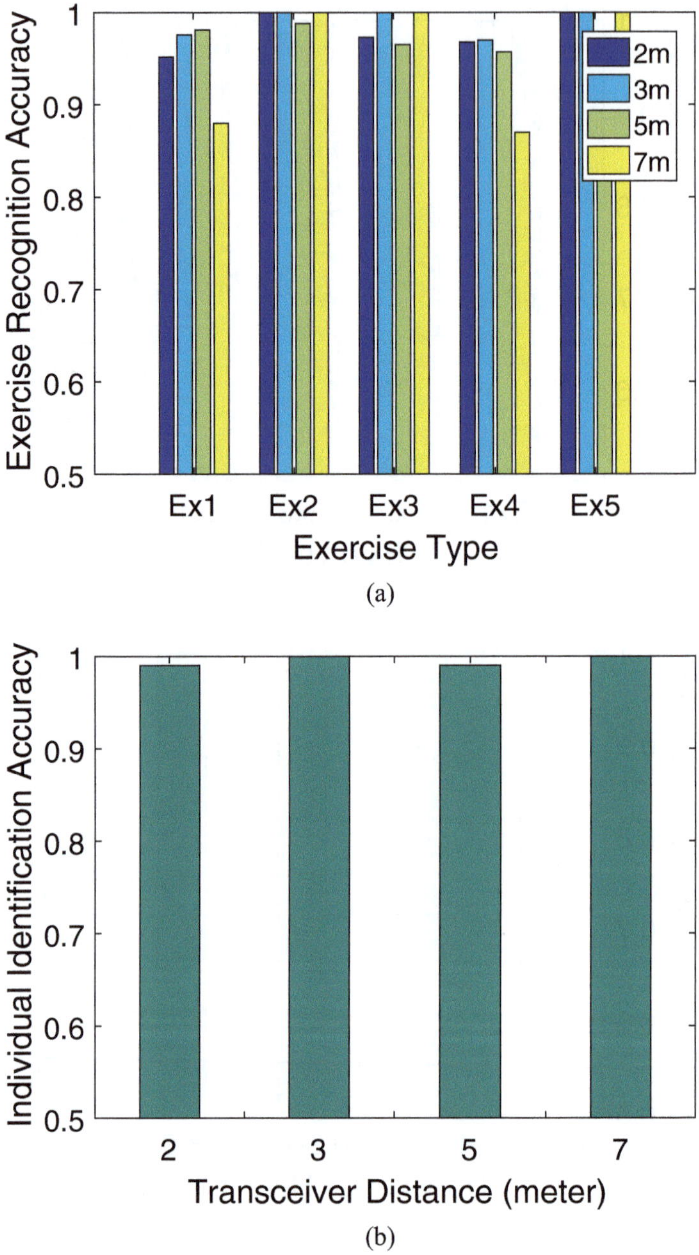

Fig. 3.13 Impact of transceiver distance on exercise recognition and individual identification. (**a**) Workout recognition. (**b**) Individual identification

3.7.6 Impact of User Location Shift

Finally, we study the impact of location shift if workout profile and testing data are collected at slightly different locations (e.g., one foot away). An opportunistic profile construction technique is adopted to build the user's workout profile at 5 different locations within a certain area, where the user deliberately changes his location when performing the same exercise. As a comparison, we also build another workout profile without opportunistic profile construction (i.e., a user's profile collected from the exact same location only). We present the experimental results for both with and without the opportunistic profile construction as shown in Fig. 3.14. Figure 3.14a reports the workout recognition results in a confusion matrix, and we observe low average recognition accuracy around 32% without opportunistic profile construction. By contrast, with the opportunistic profiles, the workout recognition results significantly improved from 32 to 92% as shown in the confusion matrix in Fig. 3.14b. This comparison further confirms the robustness of our system.

3.7.7 Performance of Different Classifiers

We further compare the DNN model with other four traditional classifiers, including k-nearest neighbors, decision tree (DT), random forest (RF) and support vector machine (SVM). Each classifier is evaluated using 10-fold cross-validation, and the parameters of each classifier are tuned to achieve the best performance. We can observe in Fig. 3.15 that the DNN-based classifier achieves the best workout recognition and individual identification accuracies among the five classifiers. As shown in Fig. 3.15a, for workout recognition, the other four classifiers have average accuracies of 87, 58, 79, 81%, respectively. And for individual identification accuracies as depicted in Fig. 3.15b, the four classification models have average accuracies of 90, 88, 83, 87%, which are less effective than the designed DNN model. Moreover, we observe that the DNN model obtains the lowest variances of 3.1 and 1.9% for workout recognition and individual identification respectively. Thus, our DNN model maintain consistent performance in the cross-validation process. This is because the linear-classifiers fail to mitigate the impacts of non-linear value variations introduced by propagation path changes. Therefore, we adopt the DNN model for both workout recognition and individual identification tasks in this work.

3.8 Conclusion

The propagation strength of waves between a transceiver pair is governed by the Fresnel zone. This zone comprises a sequence of concentric prolate ellipsoidal regions between a transmitting and receiving antenna. We designate the area within

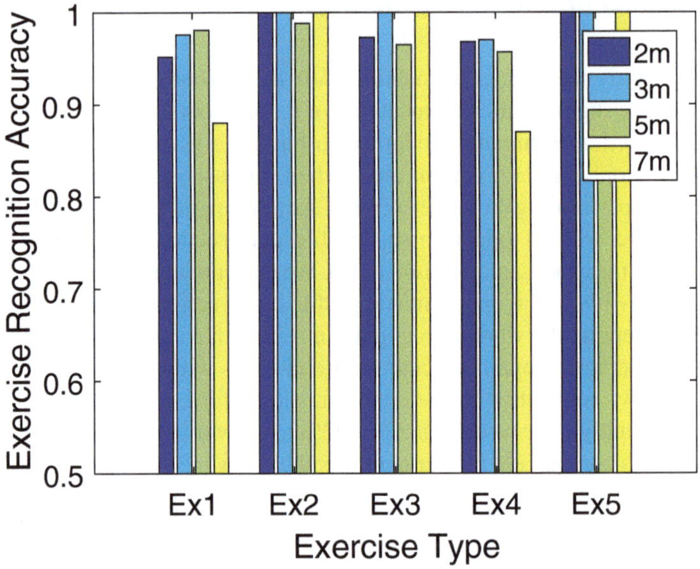

(a)

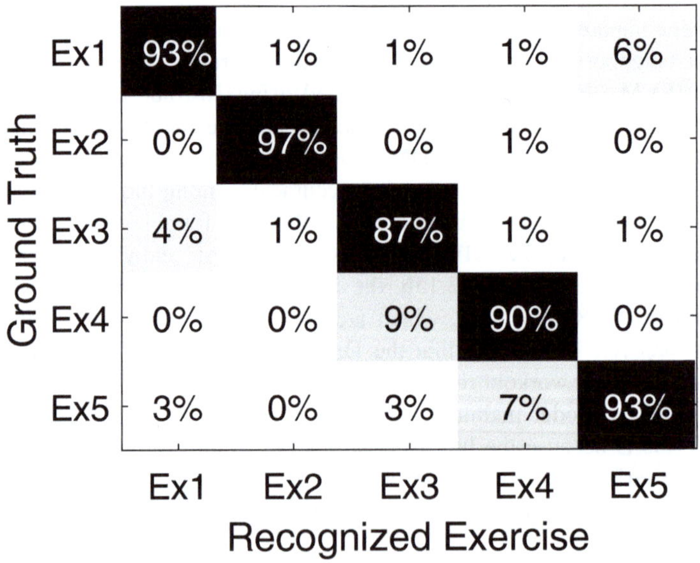

(b)

Fig. 3.14 Improvement of workout recognition accuracy with opportunistic profile construction. (**a**) Without opportunistic profiles. (**b**) With opportunistic profiles

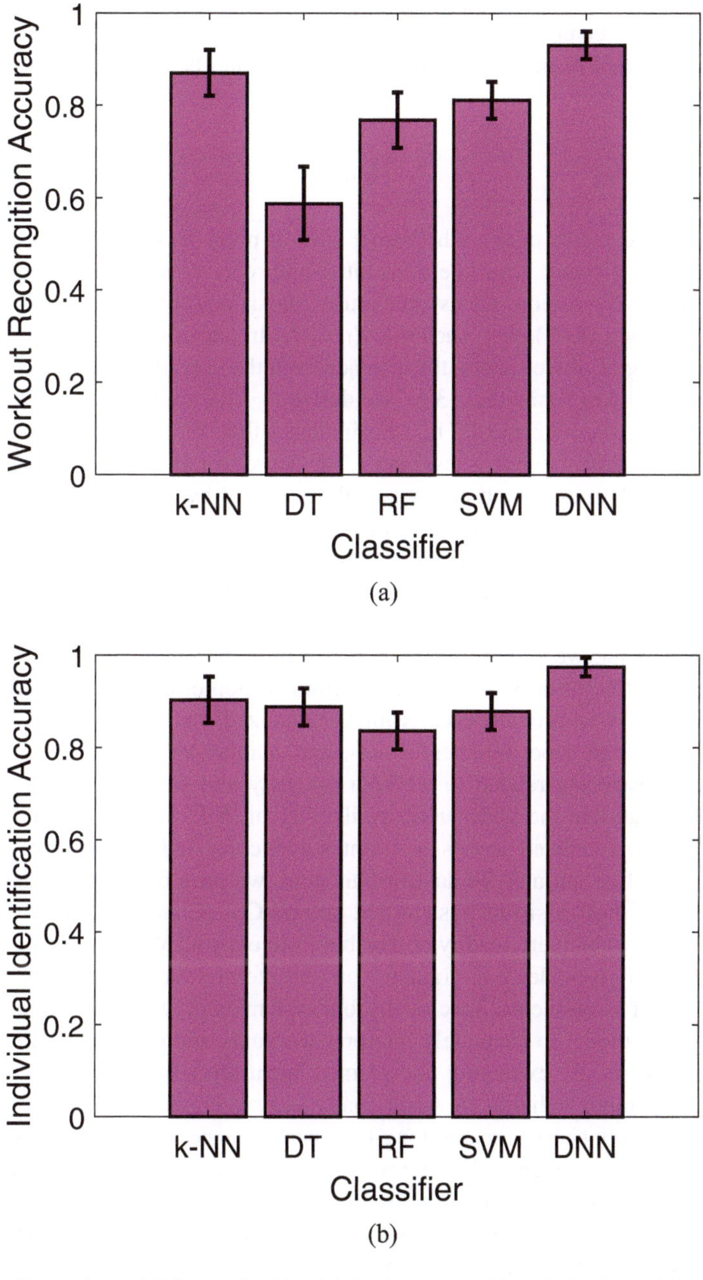

Fig. 3.15 Comparison of different classifier. (**a**) Workout recognition. (**b**) Individual identification

the 12th Fresnel zone as the *Sensitive Region*. This is because RF signal transmission between a transceiver pair predominantly occurs within the first 8–12 zones [15]. The radius of the Fresnel zone at point p can be explicitly determined by:

$$r_n = \sqrt{\frac{n\lambda d_1 d_2}{d_1 + d_2}}, \tag{3.6}$$

where r_n is the radius of the nth Fresnel zone at point p, λ is the wavelength, d_1 and d_2 are the distance from the transmitter and receiver to p, respectively. For a standard room dimension, we assume a user stands equidistant from both ends of the Line of Sight (LoS) path, such that $d_1 = d_2$. In our system deployment within common living or office spaces, the distance from the user to any device is typically between 2 and 4 m. Using Eq. (3.6), we derive r_{12} (the radius of the 12th Fresnel zone) to lie between 1.2 and 1.7 m. This indicates that, for standard room sizes, the radius of the sensitive region is less than 1.7 m. Moreover, in real-world settings such as offices and homes, which are frequently occupied by multiple individuals, the Channel State Information (CSI) dynamics related to one user's workout pattern can be influenced by the daily activities of those around them. However, our theoretical analysis on the Fresnel zone suggests that interference from nearby individuals should be minimal, provided they move outside the designated sensitive region.

In this chapter, we explore the potential of utilizing ubiquitous WiFi signals to enhance the effectiveness of exercise routines in home and office environments. Our objective is to provide users with personalized, detailed workout statistics, including workout type, number of sets, and number of repetitions, as well as dynamic assessments related to workout intensity and strength. In our research, we demonstrate that the widespread availability of WiFi signals can be leveraged to create a personalized fitness assistant suitable for individuals working from home or in office settings. To achieve this goal, we have developed a device-free personalized fitness assistant system that utilizes CSI (Channel State Information) measurements, which are readily obtainable from existing WiFi infrastructure. Our system not only provides fine-grained workout interpretation but also incorporates smart workout assessments. Specifically, our system employs a deep neural network (DNN)-based model to accurately interpret workouts and conduct comprehensive workout analysis. By extracting fine-grained latent representations, we are able to further differentiate individuals. Additionally, our system evaluates workout quality by analyzing both short-term and long-term performance, enabling users to receive valuable workout reviews. These reviews help users improve their subsequent exercises and minimize the risk of unnecessary injuries. To validate the effectiveness of our system, we conducted extensive experiments involving 20 volunteers across three typical indoor venues. The results of these experiments indicate that our system achieves high accuracy rates, with over 93% accuracy in identifying workout types and over 97% accuracy in associating individuals with their workouts, using only a single pair of WiFi transmitter and receiver. These promising outcomes suggest that our system has the potential to greatly enhance personalized fitness assistance, while also being adaptable to various application scenarios, ultimately benefiting people in their daily lives.

References

1. Adib, F., Kabelac, Z., Katabi, D., Miller, R.C.: 3d tracking via body radio reflections. In: 11th USENIX Symposium on Networked Systems Design and Implementation (USENIX NSDI), vol. 14, pp. 317–329 (2014)
2. American College of Sports Medicine, et al.: ACSM's guidelines for exercise testing and prescription. Lippincott Williams & Wilkins, Philadelphia (2013)
3. Arney, J.: You should be in pictures! experts share tips on how to produce a quality fitness video for any purpose. IDEA Fitness J. **2**(1), 86–90 (2005)
4. Bachu, R., Kopparthi, S., Adapa, B., Barkana, B.D.: Voiced/unvoiced decision for speech signals based on zero-crossing rate and energy. In: Advanced Techniques in Computing Sciences and Software Engineering, pp. 279–282. Springer (2010)
5. Bishop, C.M.: Pattern recognition. Mach. Learn. **128** (2006)
6. Çeliktutan, O., Akgul, C.B., Wolf, C., Sankur, B.: Graph-based analysis of physical exercise actions. In: ACM International Workshop on Multimedia Indexing and Information Retrieval for Healthcare (ACM MIIRH), pp. 23–32 (2013)
7. Chang, K.h., Chen, M.Y., Canny, J.: Tracking free-weight exercises. In: Proceedings of the 9th International Conference on Ubiquitous Computing (ACM UbiComp) (2007)
8. Cheng, H.T., Sun, F.T., Griss, M., Davis, P., Li, J., You, D.: Nuactiv: recognizing unseen new activities using semantic attribute-based learning. In: Proceeding of the 11th Annual International Conference on Mobile Systems, Applications, and Services (ACM Mobisys) (2013)
9. Collobert, R., Weston, J.: A unified architecture for natural language processing: Deep neural networks with multitask learning. In: Proceedings of the 25th International Conference on Machine learning, pp. 160–167. ACM (2008)
10. Ding, H., Shangguan, L., Yang, Z., Han, J., Zhou, Z., Yang, P., Xi, W., Zhao, J.: Femo: a platform for free-weight exercise monitoring with rfids. In: Proceedings of the 13th ACM Conference on Embedded Networked Sensor Systems (ACM Sensys), pp. 141–154 (2015)
11. Fitbit (2014). http://www.fitbit.com/
12. Guo, X., Jian, L., Chen, Y.: Fitcoach: virtual fitness coach empowered by wearable mobile devices. In: Proceedings of the International Conference on Computer Communications (IEEE INFOCOM) (2017)
13. Halperin, D., Hu, W., Sheth, A., Wetherall, D.: Tool release: gathering 802.11 n traces with channel state information. ACM SIGCOMM Comput. Commun. Rev. **41**(1), 53–53 (2011)
14. Halperin, D., Hu, W., Sheth, A., Wetherall, D.: Predictable 802.11 packet delivery from wireless channel measurements. ACM SIGCOMM Comput. Commun. Rev. **40**, 159–170 (2010)
15. Hristov, H.D.: Fresnal Zones in Wireless Links, Zone Plate Lenses and Antennas. Artech House, Inc., Boston (2000)
16. Lee, H., Grosse, R., Ranganath, R., Ng, A.Y.: Convolutional deep belief networks for scalable unsupervised learning of hierarchical representations. In: Proceedings of the 26th Annual International Conference on Machine Learning, pp. 609–616. ACM (2009)
17. Li, H., Chan, E.C., Guo, X., Xiao, J., Wu, K., Ni, L.M.: Wi-counter: smartphone-based people counter using crowdsourced wi-fi signal data. IEEE Trans. Human-Machine Syst. **45**(4), 442–452 (2015)

18. Liu, C., Zhang, L., Liu, Z., Liu, K., Li, X., Liu, Y.: Lasagna: towards deep hierarchical understanding and searching over mobile sensing data. In: Proceedings of the 22nd Annual International Conference on Mobile Computing and Networking (ACM MobiCom), pp. 334–347 (2016)
19. Olshausen, B.A., Field, D.J.: Sparse coding with an overcomplete basis set: a strategy employed by v1? Vision Res. **37**(23), 3311–3325 (1997)
20. Pu, Q., Gupta, S., Gollakota, S., Patel, S.: Whole-home gesture recognition using wireless signals. In: Proceedings of the 19th Annual International Conference on Mobile Computing and Networking (ACM MobiCom), pp. 27–38 (2013)
21. Sadanand, S., Corso, J.J.: Action bank: a high-level representation of activity in video. In: IEEE Conference on Computer Vision and Pattern Recognition (IEEE CVPR), pp. 1234–1241 (2012)
22. Sarikaya, R., Hinton, G.E., Deoras, A.: Application of deep belief networks for natural language understanding. IEEE/ACM Trans. Audio Speech Language Process. (TASLP) **22**(4), 778–784 (2014)
23. Socher, R., Bengio, Y., Manning, C.: Deep learning for nlp. Tutorial at Association of Computational Logistics (ACL), 2012, and North American Chapter of the Association of Computational Linguistics (NAACL) (2013)
24. Su, C.J., Chiang, C.Y., Huang, J.Y.: Kinect-enabled home-based rehabilitation system using dynamic time warping and fuzzy logic. Appl. Soft Comput. **22**, 652–666 (2014)
25. Sun, Y., Wang, X., Tang, X.: Deep learning face representation from predicting 10,000 classes. In: Proceedings of the IEEE Conference on Computer Vision and Pattern Recognition, pp. 1891–1898 (2014)
26. Vincent, P., Larochelle, H., Lajoie, I., Bengio, Y., Manzagol, P.A.: Stacked denoising autoencoders: learning useful representations in a deep network with a local denoising criterion. J. Mach. Learn. Res. **11**, 3371–3408 (2010)
27. Wang, N., Yeung, D.Y.: Learning a deep compact image representation for visual tracking. In: Advances in Neural Information Processing Systems, pp. 809–817 (2013)
28. Wang, Y., Liu, J., Chen, Y., Gruteser, M., Yang, J., Liu, H.: E-eyes: device-free location-oriented activity identification using fine-grained wifi signatures. In: Proceedings of the 20th Annual International Conference on Mobile Computing and Networking (ACM MobiCom), pp. 617–628 (2014)
29. Wang, W., Liu, A.X., Shahzad, M., Ling, K., Lu, S.: Understanding and modeling of wifi signal based human activity recognition. In: Proceedings of the 21st Annual International Conference on Mobile Computing and Networking (ACM MobiCom), pp. 65–76 (2015)
30. Wu, J., Osuntogun, A., Choudhury, T., Philipose, M., Rehg, J.M.: A scalable approach to activity recognition based on object use. In: 11th International Conference on Computer Vision (IEEE ICCV), pp. 1–8 (2007)
31. Xie, J., Xu, L., Chen, E.: Image denoising and inpainting with deep neural networks. In: Advances in Neural Information Processing Systems, pp. 341–349 (2012)

Chapter 4
Multi-person Fitness Assistance via Millimeter Wave

The next generation of WiFi incorporates integrated millimeter-wave technology, which leverages high-frequency radio waves in the millimeter range to enable wireless data transmission. The key advantages of mmWave over traditional WiFi frequencies (such as 2.4 and 5 GHz) are its wide bandwidth and directional characteristics. Recently, there is a growing trend in employing mmWave signals for fitness monitoring, driven by their wide bandwidth and directional characteristics. In this chapter, we present a millimeter-wave-based fitness monitoring system that offers personalized and environment-independent monitoring with reduced training requirements in a multi-person scenario. To address limited training data, we employ a GAN-assisted method that achieves satisfactory performance. Additionally, we develop a domain adaptation training framework to enhance system robustness and enable deployment in new environments with minimal training efforts. Our system utilizes a unique Spatial-Temporal Heatmap feature for personalized workout recognition and incorporates a point-cloud-based method for concurrent multi-person workout monitoring. Extensive experiments demonstrate that our system achieves high accuracy in workout recognition and user identification.

The rest of the chapter is organized as follows. We present a research background in Sect. 4.1 and discuss related work in Sect. 4.2. In Sect. 4.3, we provide a fundamental study of mmWave radar and its feasibility for fitness monitoring. We then proceed to present the design of the multi-person fitness assistant system via millimeter wave in Sect. 4.4. In Sect. 4.5, we describe the use of Generative Adversarial Networks (GAN) to reduce training efforts. Next, we elaborate the system implementation and provide system evaluation in Sect. 4.6. Finally, we discuss and conclude our work in Sect. 4.7.

X. Guo et al., *Mobile Technologies for Smart Healthcare System Design*,
Wireless Networks, https://doi.org/10.1007/978-3-031-57345-3_4

4.1 Background

Nowadays, many people perform physical exercises regularly at home for convenience, safety, and flexibility. Though there are various at-home workout and fitness programs available to help users achieve certain fitness goals, the lack of professional guidance and monitoring can make this process less effective. For example, you might not be able to do the exercises in correct positions and forms; your workout is not consistent or imbalanced between aerobic and strength training. Therefore, it is important to have an in-home fitness monitoring system that can track the exercise process of users and give them useful suggestions.

Traditional camera-based fitness monitoring may raise serious privacy concerns [3, 7], while sensor-based methods require users to wear dedicated devices [1, 16]. Some researchers propose to utilize WiFi signals for non-intrusive fitness monitoring [8, 27]. However WiFi signals are sensitive to interference and surrounding environment changes. In recent years, millimeter wave (mmWave) signals have emerged for activity recognition since they enable higher-resolution sensing given their short wavelengths and high bandwidths. In addition, mmWave has already been integrated into the next-generation WiFi standards (i.e., IEEE 802.11ad). For example, human skeleton systems are proposed to capture human postures [24, 31, 33]. However, these systems require extra cameras (e.g., Microsoft Kinect) to provide accurate joint locations. Moreover, some activity recognition systems have shown satisfying performance for one-person scenarios [23, 26, 29]. Since, in reality, multiple persons may be present in a shared space, a system suitable for concurrent workout scenarios is desired for fitness monitoring.

Although mmWave has the potential to offer higher signal resolution comparing to traditional RF-based approaches, mmWave-based solutions still face technical challenges and obstacles for real deployment. First, existing mmWave-based methods need to collect enough amount of data for training machine learning models up to a satisfactory level of accuracy [2, 23, 31]. For example, they require users to repeat the activity moves many times. This makes it inconvenient and time-consuming for practical usage. Second, the trained machine learning models are environment-specific and re-training processes are required before they can be applied to a new environment [18, 22, 24]. Third, even in the same environment, users can work out in different spots. These small changes in locations can have a significant impact on the system performance [14, 26]. In summary, it is essential to develop a multi-person fitness monitoring system robust of environmental variations with light efforts in training data collection.

Toward this end, we design and develop a mmWave-based personalized fitness monitoring system using only a single COTS mmWave device. The system integrates modules of workout recognition, user identification, multi-user monitoring, and training effort reduction. Specifically, our system records mmWave signals reflected from human bodies and captures fine-grained workout information, such as workout types, repetitions, and participants. For workout recognition and user identification, a new spatial-temporal heatmap is designed to capture workout dynamics using various activity characteristics (i.e., velocity, range of movements, and time duration). For multi-person monitoring, we utilize a clustering-based method to construct a spatial-temporal heatmap for each user based on the reflected signals. We then develop deep neural network models to extract unique high-dimensional features from the heatmaps to perform the workout and user identification tasks.

In addition, we develop a generative adversarial network (GAN) to synthesize a large number of virtual workout segments based on a small number of segments collected from real users. By adding these virtual segments to training data sets, our system achieves better system performance. Furthermore, because in practice there are variations in users' face orientations, locations, and environments (e.g., different rooms, furniture placements, etc.), we define these types of variations as domains and develop a domain adaptation framework to learn the domain-independent feature representations to improve the robustness of our system. We also design a method to mitigate environmental impacts and eliminate static components in the mmWave signals. This lays the groundwork for adapting the system to new environments.

The contributions of this chapter are summarized as follows. We design and implement a fitness monitoring system using a single COTS mmWave device. The designed system integrates workout recognition, user identification, multi-user monitoring, and training effort reduction modules. To reduce training efforts, we develop a domain adaptation framework that mitigates the impacts caused by domain characteristics embedded in mmWave signals, thus reducing the amount of training data needed from different domains. We also employ a GAN-assisted method to achieve better workout recognition and user identification when only limited training data from the same domain is available. For personalized workout recognition, we explore a unique spatial-temporal heatmap feature that integrates multiple workout features such as range of movement, velocity, and time duration. Additionally, we develop a clustering-based method to derive a spatial-temporal heatmap for each user, enabling multi-person workout monitoring. We implement a prototype of the system and evaluate its performance using 14 types of full-body workouts and over 7000 workout segments from various real-world scenarios. Our system achieves average accuracies of 97% in workout recognition and 91% in user identification with small training data (e.g. 10 repetitions per workout type). When training is performed with only one repetition per workout type, the accuracies moderately drop to 85% in workout recognition and 81% in user identification.

4.2 Related Work

In general, activity recognition and fitness monitoring systems can be classified into three categories: camera-based [3, 25], sensor-based [1, 16],and radio-frequency (RF) signal-based [8, 26]. In this part, we will review existing works and compare them with the designed mmWave-based fitness monitoring system.

A couple of camera-based systems have been proposed to recognize human activities and perform fitness monitoring [3, 7, 25]. These works use cameras to capture images or videos and apply image-processing algorithms to extract motions or user identities. However, camera-based methods may raise privacy concerns. To address this weakness, sensor-based systems have been developed [1, 9, 16]. These works explore various non-intrusive sensors like gyrometer [9], ECG [16] or FSR sensor [1] to collect different types of signals for further analysis. However, sensor-based approaches require users to wear sensors or other devices, which is inconvenient for senior people or during complex activities.

To overcome the above limitations, researchers recently propose to exploit RF-based methods (e.g., WiFi and mmWave). WiFi-based approaches [8, 27] use off-the-shelf WiFi devices to infer activities and users' identifies. However, being easily influenced by surrounding environments remains the main limitation. Compared with WiFi signal, mmWave has been proven to be robust for activity recognition due to the antenna directionality and stability. Some researchers propose to build human skeleton systems to capture human postures [24, 31–34]. However, these systems require special cameras (e.g., Microsoft Kinect) to provide accurate joint locations. Extra devices requirements and privacy concerns might limit the widespread deployments of these approaches for in-home fitness monitoring. Besides, many activity recognition works have shown satisfying performance for single-user scenarios. [10, 12, 22, 23, 26, 28, 29]. However, multiple family members may perform workouts simultaneously in a shared space. Thus, a system that works in concurrent scenarios is desired for fitness monitoring. To address this weakness, researchers propose approaches [2, 11, 14, 18, 30] that could track multiple people simultaneously. However, these approaches usually require users to repeat dozens of times (e.g., 30 times) of the same gesture or activity in the training stage, which is time-consuming and labor-intensive to build a module including multiple types of workouts. Furthermore, training and testing data might be different in terms of people's orientations, locations, and environments, thus requiring significant training efforts. In addition, it is still desired to have a system that could identify people along with activities to provide personalized fitness monitoring. Thus, existing mmWave-based approaches are not suitable for in-home fitness monitoring.

Compared with existing work, our system enables low-effort personalized fitness monitoring using a single COTS mmWave device. We integrate multiple modules including workout recognition, user identification, multi-user monitoring, and training effort reduction into a single system. We develop a domain adaptation framework to reduce the efforts of training data collection from different domains and also develop a GAN-assisted method to achieve better performance. Furthermore, we design unique features to enable personalized workout recognition and develop a clustering-based method for multi-user monitoring.

4.3 Millimeter Wave Fundamental and Preliminaries

4.3.1 mmWave Radar Principle

The millimeter-wave (mmWave) radar system is a critical technology employed for detecting and tracking objects using frequency-modulated continuous-wave (FMCW) signals. The particular operating range of these radar systems corresponds to the millimeter wavelength, enabling them to transmit and receive signals within the millimeter range, as documented by [21]. The central function of the mmWave radar system is the emission of distinctive signals termed as 'chirps.' A chirp is characterized as a sinusoidal wave, the frequency of which undergoes a linear increase over time. This property makes chirps highly beneficial for radar applications as they allow precise determination of range, velocity, and other attributes of detected objects. Each chirp's properties can be defined using three primary parameters: bandwidth (B), duration (Tc), and slope (S). The bandwidth of a chirp is the frequency range that it covers, which directly influences the resolution of the radar system. In contrast, the duration (Tc) refers to the temporal length of a single chirp cycle. The slope of a chirp, on the other hand, delineates the rate at which the frequency of the chirp increases linearly over time. It is an important parameter that affects the separation between targets in the range and Doppler domains. Post transmission, the radar system waits for the return of these signals as they bounce off objects within the radar's coverage area. The returned chirp, upon interception, is then mixed with a reference copy of the original transmitted signal. The mixing process involves combining the properties of the two signals to produce a resultant waveform known as the Intermediate Frequency (IF) signal, as explicated by [13]. The IF signal is instrumental in radar applications as it carries crucial information about the detected object, including its range and relative speed. By processing and analyzing this IF signal, the radar system can extract valuable insights about the surroundings, contributing significantly to applications like autonomous driving, weather radar, and air traffic control among others.

To facilitate fitness monitoring via mmWave, we first need to understand how a target affects the IF signal. A target object in front of the radar produces an IF signal with a constant frequency tone of $2dS/c$. The distance between the target and radar can be calculated as $\frac{f_{IF} \cdot c}{2 \cdot S}$, where c is the speed of light. Besides, the target with a moving speed v should have different phases across two consecutive chirps. The phase difference ω measured across two consecutive chirps can be used to estimate the velocity of the object through $\frac{\lambda \cdot \omega}{4\pi \cdot T_c}$, where λ is the wavelength. Furthermore, different distances from the object to different antennas on the radar result in phase differences. The measured phase difference ω across different antennas can be used to estimate the AoA of the object using $\sin^{-1}\left(\frac{\lambda \cdot \omega}{2\pi l}\right)$, where l is the distance between neighboring antennas.

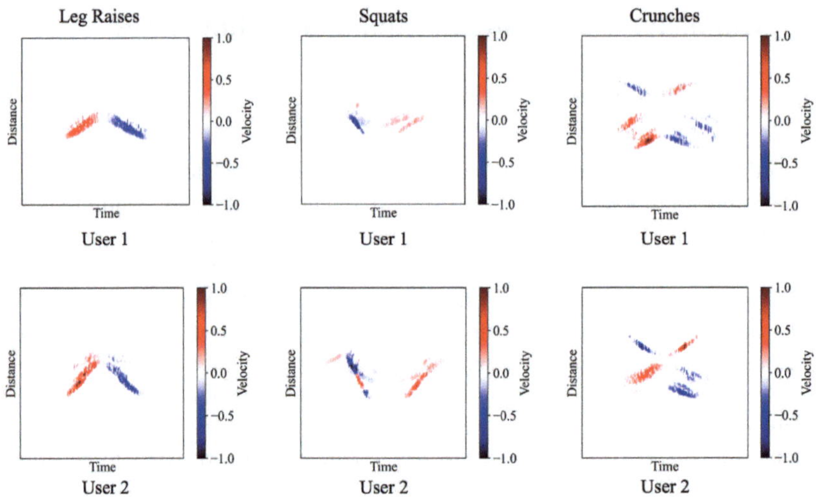

Fig. 4.1 Spatial-temporal heatmaps of three different workouts of two users

4.3.2 Feasibility Study of Using mmWave for Fitness Monitoring

To demonstrate the feasibility of fitness monitoring via mmWave, we conduct experiments with two participants performing different types of workouts (e.g., leg raises, squats, and crunches) in front of a mmWave device (i.e., AWR1642), respectively. Although we can measure the distance, velocity from mmWave signals separately, integrating multiple workout features to represent human dynamics is important since it exhibits the differences among various workouts more clearly. In this research, we develop spatial-temporal heatmaps to enable personalized fitness monitoring. As shown in Fig. 4.1, in a spatial-temporal heatmap, the horizontal axis represents the time duration of a workout repetition while the vertical axis represents the range of movement. The velocity is represented by color. We observe that spatial-temporal heatmaps of different workouts present different patterns, which demonstrate the feasibility of workout recognition. Moreover, comparing the first line and second line of Fig. 4.1, we also observe that when different people perform the same workout, spatial-temporal heatmaps would be different due to people's various heights, strengths, and figures. This observation confirms the feasibility of using the designed heatmaps for personalized workout fitness monitoring.

4.4 Multi-person Fitness Sensing System Design

The main goal of this work is to perform personalized workout monitoring by examining the dynamics of mmWave signals. As shown in Fig. 4.2, our system takes as input the mmWave signals reflected from human body. It first performs signal

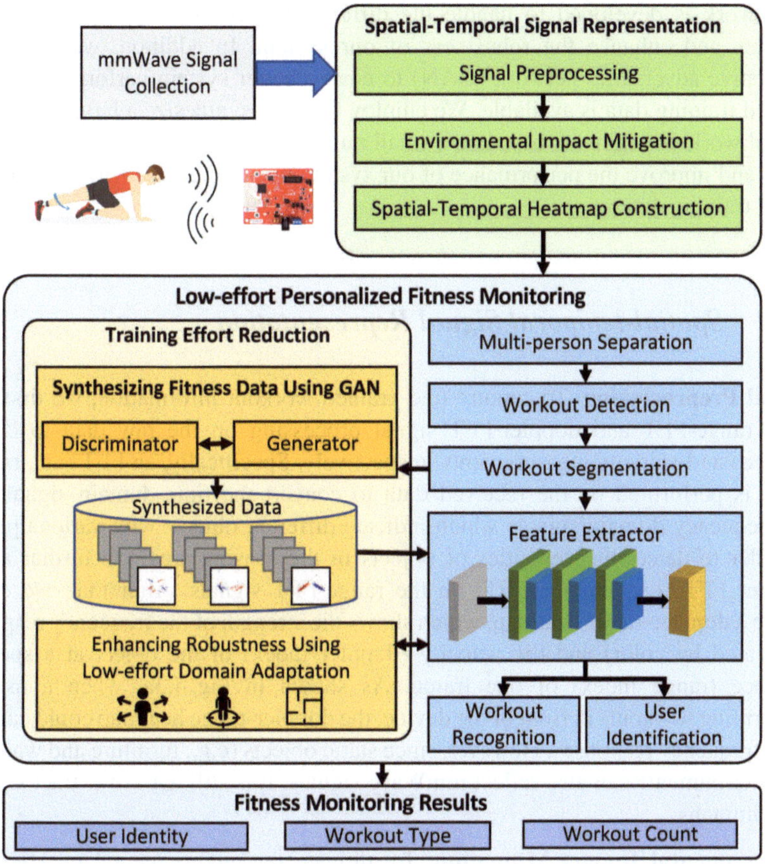

Fig. 4.2 System overview of multi-person fitness assistance via millimeter wave

processing to derive the velocity, distance, and AoA information of the users. Then, the system mitigates the impact from environments by subtracting signals reflected off static objects (i.e., tables and walls). To aggregate the spatial, temporal, and velocity features of human activities, we construct spatial-temporal heatmaps. Such signal representation integrates different activity characteristics (i.e., velocity, range of movements, and time duration) that facilitate both workout recognition and user identification. For multi-user monitoring, we utilize a clustering-based method to construct a spatial-temporal heatmap for each user based on the reflected signals. To detect workout activities from other daily activities, we design a workout detection method based on the repetitive velocity pattern of workouts in time domain.

We develop deep learning models to perform workout recognition and user identification, respectively. An extractor is used to learn feature representations, which amplifies the distinctive workout or user characteristics. A classifier is then utilized to identify workout type or user identity. Furthermore, a domain adaptation framework is developed to handle the differences between training and testing datasets and enhance the robustness of our system. In addition, we develop a generative adversarial network (GAN) to enable better system performance when limited training data is available. We employ GAN to synthesize a large number of virtual workout segments based on a small number of segments collected from real users and improve the performance of our system by adding these virtual segments to the training dataset.

4.4.1 Spatial-temporal Signal Representation

Signal Preprocessing To capture fine-grained workout information, we first perform range-FFT and doppler-FFT signal processing on the raw data to derive distance and velocity measurements, respectively. Specifically, an FFT (i.e., range-FFT) is performed on the received data to convert the time domain signal into the frequency domain signals which indicate different objects with various peaks. In order to detect the velocities of objects in the sensing area, we further apply another FFT (i.e., doppler-FFT) on the range-FFT signals. After that, we could derive a doppler-range heatmap, which shows the strength of the frequency response (indicated by color) and the velocity (doppler index) of the object at a specific distance (range index) of one frame. As shown in Fig. 4.3a, when a user is performing workouts in front of the device, the doppler-range heatmap could capture high-frequency responses. However, since static objects (e.g., furniture and walls) in the environments can also reflect mmWave signals, it is still hard to extract signals from humans.

Environmental Impact Mitigation To mitigate the environmental interference, we develop an environmental impact mitigation method by filtering out non-moving objects in doppler-range domain. Specifically, when there is no user performing workouts in the detected area, we observe that the doppler-range heatmap of the static objects (e.g., walls and furniture) remains consistent over time as shown in Fig. 4.3b. This motivates us to mitigate static impact by subtracting the time-invariant frequency responses. Specifically, we collect mmWave signals in a static environment for a short period (e.g., 1 min) to estimate the time-invariant frequency response from static objects. We further eliminate noise signals by removing frequency responses with low intensity from the dopper-range domain based on an empirical threshold. Through these procedures, as shown in Fig. 4.4a, it is clear to see the frequency responses caused by human activities in the denoised doppler-range heatmap.

Spatial-Temporal Heatmap Construction Although doppler-range heatmaps could capture velocity information in different ranges, it is insufficient to describe the process of the workout, because it does not contain temporal information, such as the time duration of each repetition and the velocity variations in time domain.

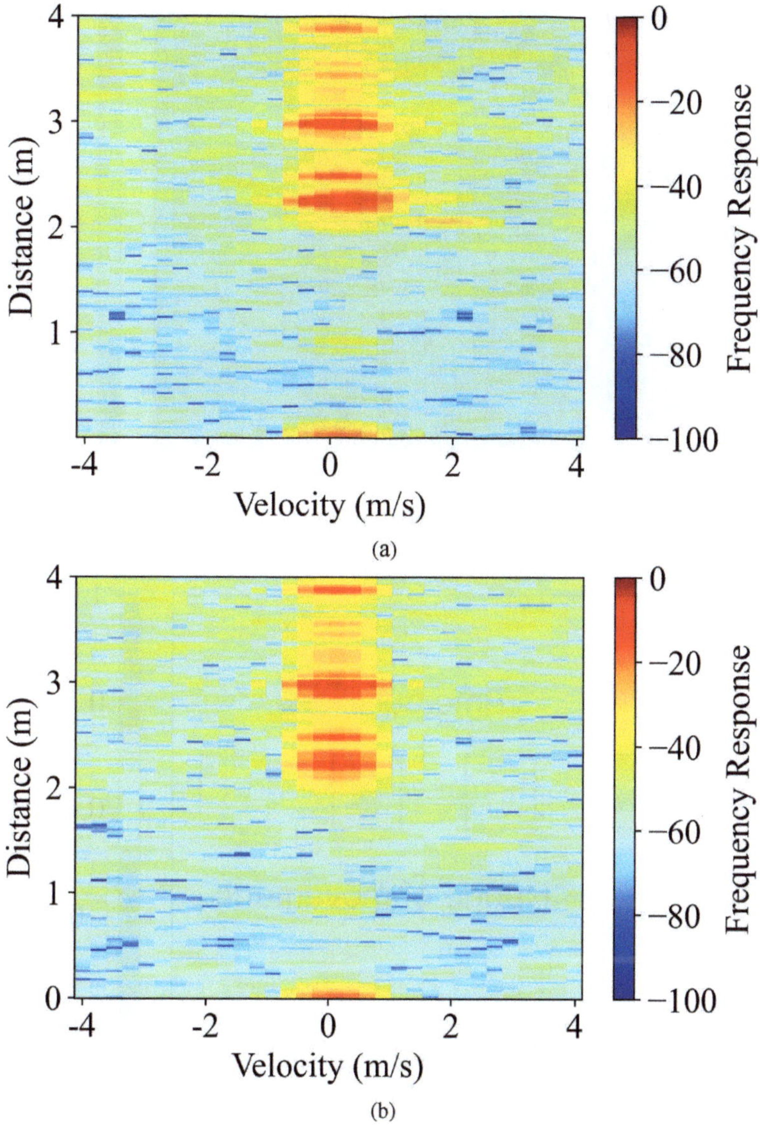

Fig. 4.3 (**a**) Doppler-range heatmap when one user is performing workout in the detection area; (**b**) Doppler-range heatmap when no user is in the detection area

To integrate multi-dimensional features, we propose to construct spatial-temporal heatmaps. Specifically, we accumulate the velocity of every distance in every doppler-range heatmap together as follows:

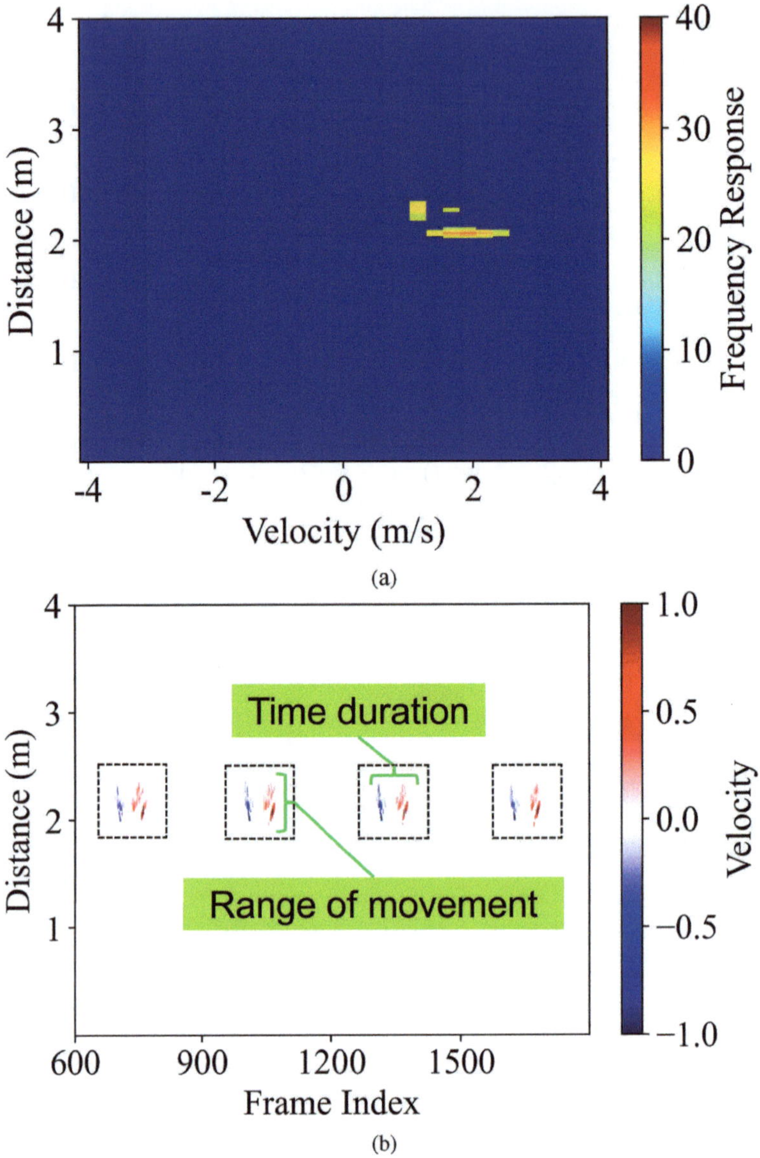

Fig. 4.4 (**a**) Doppler-range heatmap after environmental impact mitigation; (**b**) Spatial-temporal heatmap of four repetitions

$$V_{q,t} = \sum_{p=1}^{D} (I_{p,q,t}) \times v_{p,t},\ p \in [1, D],\ q \in [1, R], \tag{4.1}$$

where $I_{p,q,t}$ is the intensity of a frequency response in the doppler-range heatmap, p is the doppler index, q represents the range index, and t is the frame index. $v_{p,t}$ is the velocity corresponding to a doppler index p in frame t. Then we normalize the derived $V_{q,t}$ and transfer the original instantaneous velocity-distance relationship to a more comprehensive spatial-temporal heatmap which describes the process of a workout as shown in Fig. 4.4b.

4.4.2 Clustering-based Separation of Multiple Users

Multiple family members may perform workouts together in a shared space. In such cases, our system needs to be able to monitor multiple people's workouts concurrently using a single device. This is challenging as the mmWave signals reflected from different peoples might be mixed. We take two users' concurrent workouts as an example. When two people are performing workouts at the same distance to the mmWave device, the reflected signals from each person are hard to be differentiated in the range domain, because of the same measurements in distance. Thus, it is difficult to separate each user's workouts based on their distance in the spatial-temporal heatmap. Furthermore, when users are performing workouts at the same time, it would be even harder to separate different users' workouts because of the overlapped spatial-temporal heatmaps of two users.

In developing a method to separate the reflected signals from different users, we find that when people perform workouts, each people should have their own space to allow every part of the body to move adequately. This makes the reflected signals from different people separable in the two-dimensional spatial Cartesian coordinate system. Based on this idea, in this section, we develop a clustering-based method to achieve multiple people fitness monitoring based on different users' spatial information as shown in Fig. 4.5. Specifically, we generate the point cloud

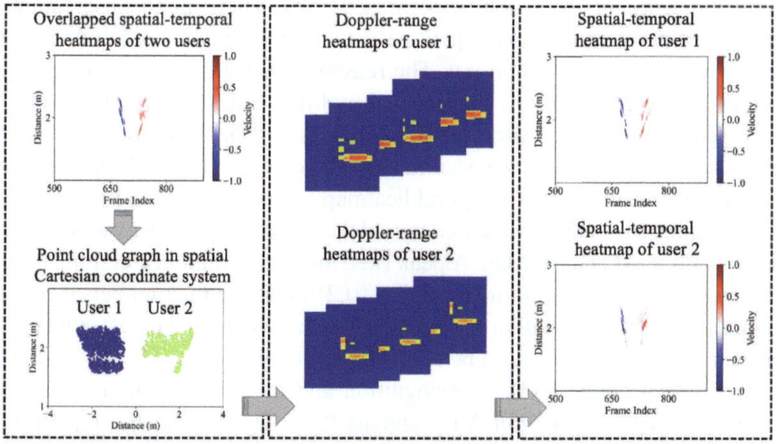

Fig. 4.5 The flow of multi-user separation

graph in the two-dimensional spatial Cartesian coordinate system via applying an FFT (angle-FFT) on the doppler-FFT signals. In particular, given a point in the doppler-range domain with range index q, doppler index p, measured distance d, and AoA (θ), taking the position of the device as the origin, we could derive the spatial coordinate of the point as follows:

$$
\begin{aligned}
x_{(p,q)} &= d_{(p,q)} \times \sin\theta_{(p,q)} \\
y_{(p,q)} &= d_{(p,q)} \times \cos\theta_{(p,q)},
\end{aligned}
\tag{4.2}
$$

where x and y are x-axis and y-axis coordinate, respectively.

We accumulate the point cloud graphs of every frame in a sliding window (i.e., 10 s) and separate the accumulated point clouds into different clusters via an unsupervised clustering method (i.e., DBSCAN). It detects the number of users by counting the number of clusters in the detected area. When more than one cluster (the number of points in each cluster should be more than an empirical threshold P_{max}) are detected in the area, our system confirms the existence of multiple users. Next, for each cluster, we map all points in the cluster back to the doppler-range domain based on Eq. (4.2). A spatial-temporal heatmap for each user can be derived based on the doppler-range heatmap of every frame in the sliding window using Eq. (4.1). We note that this point cloud-based method could also be applied in more complex scenarios with more than 2 users since multiple users' reflected signals can still be detected and separated in the spatial Cartesian coordinate system.

4.4.3 Exercise Pattern Segmentation and Clustering

After constructing spatial-temporal heatmaps for every user, we focus on distinguishing the workout from non-workout activities. There is an observation that workout activities usually have repetitive patterns in the spatial-temporal domain while non-workout activities do not. The reason is that fitness activities consist of consistent motions that usually be repeated multiple times. Based on the observation, we propose to detect workouts by searching for the repetitive patterns via a sliding window. Specifically, we accumulate the velocities from all the distances in a frame to transfer the spatial-temporal heatmap to one-dimensional data. Then, an auto-correlation-based method is used to find the repeating pattern by comparing the similarity with itself at a time lag. A peak (i.e., local maximum) detection algorithm is adopted with an empirical threshold (i.e., 0.2) to derive the number of peaks N. The workout is detected within the specific sliding window (i.e., 10 s) when N is larger than N_{min}. We set N_{min} to be 5 in our prototype system [4].

To facilitate accurate workout recognition and user identification, we need to determine the segments of mmWave signals that only contain the repetitions of workouts. In this section, we determine each workout repetition according to their time duration and range of movement in the spatial-temporal heatmap. Specifically, we utilize a threshold to set the points in the heatmap with a low absolute velocity to zero. The threshold is selected from empirical studies. Then, we use DBSCAN to separate the points into different clusters based on the coordinates of the points in the heatmap. To segment each repetition more accurately, we design a dynamic segmentation algorithm that determines the 2D window size of each repetition according to its time duration and range of movement in the spatial-temporal heatmap. As shown in Fig. 4.4b, for each repetition, we find the coordinates of minimum and maximum points in the frame-distance plane. Then, we derive the window size based on the differences between the coordinates of the extreme points. We scale up the size of the window by a constant (i.e., 1.2) which is empirically determined to ensure robustness.

4.5 Reducing Training Effort

4.5.1 Reducing Training Effort in Cross-domain Deployment

To reduce the training efforts for cross-domain deployments and improve the robustness of our system, we develop a domain adaptation framework. This framework uses the spatial-temporal segments obtained from previous processes as input. The data is first converted into a feature extractor. Based on the feature representations, a classifier is developed to predict the workout or corresponding user. To mitigate domain characteristics (e.g., user's face orientation, location, and environment) embedded in feature representations, a discriminator that can differentiate domains is developed to help optimize the feature extractor. By optimizing the feature extractor to "fool" domain discriminator but also support workout/user classifier, the framework can facilitate the deployments across different domains and improve robustness. Figure 4.6 shows the structure of the proposed domain adaptation framework.

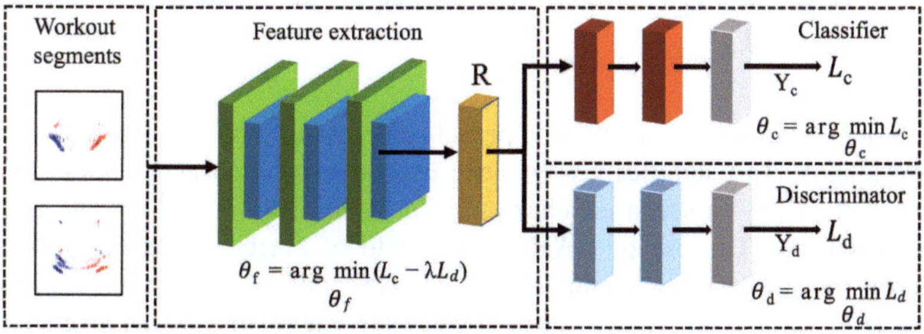

Fig. 4.6 Domain adaptation framework for training effort reduction

Designing Workout Recognition and User Identification Model The feature extractor has three convolutional layers, each with a 3×3 filter and a ReLU activation function. Each convolutional layer is followed by a max-pooling layer with a stride of 2 and a filter size of 2×2 to downsample and reduce data redundancy. After the process of 3 rounds of up-sampling and down-sampling, a 64-dimension feature map is obtained. Then, a flatten layer is integrated to reduce the feature map into a one-dimension array. Given an input data D, the feature extractor produces feature representations $R = F(D, \Theta_f)$, where F represents the feature extractor and Θ_f represents its trainable parameters. Based on the derived feature representation R, a neural network consisting of two dense layers is followed to classify the inputs into several classes (e.g., different types of workouts). We train two classifiers with same structure to differentiate workouts and user identities, respectively. Given the input representation R, the classifier predicts the label as Y_c. We optimize the classifier by minimizing the cross-entropy loss between the ground truth $\tilde{Y_c}$ and the predicted label Y_c as $L_c = L_{CE}\left(Y_c, \tilde{Y_c}\right)$, where L_{CE} represent the cross-entropy loss function.

Domain Adaptation Training To reduce the amount of training data collected from different domains, we use domain adaptation training [6] to transfer our system to new domains. Specifically, we develop a domain discriminator to make the feature representations similar between different domains. The proposed domain discriminator consists of two dense layers. It takes the feature representations R as inputs and predicts the domain labels Y_d (e.g., original environment or a new environment). We optimize the discriminator with the cross-entropy loss between the ground truth domain $\tilde{Y_d}$ and the predicted domain Y_d as $L_d = L_{CE}\left(Y_d, \tilde{Y}_d'\right)$. To make the extracted features domain-independent, we design an adversarial loss as $L_{adv} = L_c - \lambda L_d$, where L_c is the classification loss and L_d is the discriminator loss. We set domain loss L_d to negative since we would like to train the feature extractor to maximize the domain loss. The factor λ is selected to control the balance between the transferability and distinguishability of the extracted features.

4.5.2 *Reducing Training Effort Using Generative Adversarial Networks*

In this part, we deveop a novel approach employing a Generative Adversarial Network (GAN) to significantly enhance user identification and workout recognition, particularly in scenarios characterized by limited domain-specific training data availability. The use of GANs in the field of machine learning presents a powerful tool to generate synthetic data, thereby addressing data scarcity issues. Generative Adversarial Networks have been widely applied across a diverse range of applications, given their potent ability to model and mimic complex data distributions. From human identification [20] to sophisticated healthcare systems

[5, 17], GANs have consistently demonstrated promising results, extending beyond traditional expectations and setting new benchmarks in the respective fields. One of the key features of GANs is their capacity for synthetic data generation, significantly reducing the required effort for model training. In our work, the primary focus is to exploit the capabilities of GANs to augment the training data specifically for workout recognition tasks. With the assistance of GANs, we aim to generate additional synthetic data instances that are representative of different types of workouts. This approach will considerably enrich our training dataset, thereby contributing to the development of a robust user identification and workout recognition system, especially in scenarios where data availability from the same domain is limited.

Workout Data Generation Using GAN The GAN used in our work is composed of two sub-networks: a generator G and a discriminator D. As shown in Fig. 4.7, G aims to learn the distribution of the real workout segments to synthesize virtual data. D tries to discriminate whether a workout is real or synthesized. G and D compete with each other to achieve their goals, which leading to a two-player mini-max game. The overall value function $V(D, G)$ is defined by:

$$\min_{G} \max_{D} V(D, G) = \log(D(x)) + \log(1 - D(G(n))), \tag{4.3}$$

where x represents a real workout, n represents a noise vector. $G(n)$ is synthesized workout generated by G. $D(\cdot)$ is discriminator's estimation that the data is a real workout. The basic training process of GAN is described as follows: G tries to maximize the probability that a synthesized workout is discriminated as real by minimizing the generator loss function $L_G = -\log(D(G(n)))$. On the other hand, D tries to maximize the probability that the real and virtual workout are

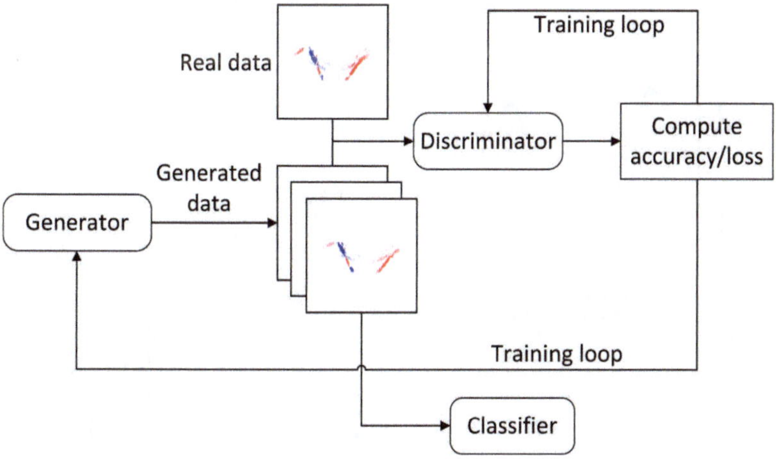

Fig. 4.7 Structure of the GAN for workouts generation

classified correctly by maximizing the discriminator loss $L_D = -\log(D(x)) - \log(1 - D(G(n)))$. G and D are trained in turn to optimize each other by updating parameters of their networks. The final state is a Nash equilibrium where the generated workouts are similar to the real ones, and the discriminator fails to identify whether the workouts are real or not.

GAN Implementation and Visualization In the system, both G and D are implemented by convolutional neural networks (CNN). G has 5 transpose convolutional layers. D has 6 convolutional layers followed by a flatten layer. After the competing of the generator and the discriminator, our GAN network eventually generate a large number of high-quality synthesized workouts. Even when users only perform a small number of repetitions in real-life scenarios, with the assistance of the generated workout dataset, the system can be well-trained offline and thus guarantee a good workout recognition and user identification performance online. To give an overall evaluation of the quality of the GAN-generated workouts, we generate virtual workouts based on a small number of real workouts (i.e., one repetition per workout type). Then we utilize t-SNE [15] to visualize the similarity between real and GAN-generated workouts. Specifically, GAN-generated and real workouts are firstly converted by the feature extractor. Then, t-SNE is applied to the extracted high-dimensional feature representations for dimension reduction. Finally, the feature embedding of each workout is obtained and illustrated in a 2-D plane as shown in Fig. 4.8. We observe that the feature embedding of the

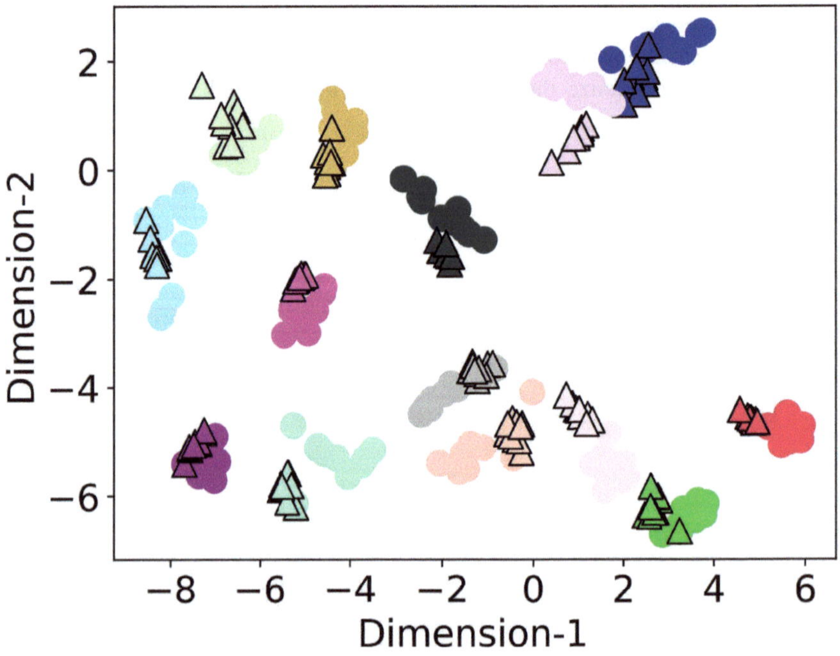

Fig. 4.8 Distributions of real (circle) and generated (triangle) workouts. Each color represents one workout type

GAN-generated repetitions overlap with the real ones from the same workout type but have no overlap with those from different types. This indicates that the GAN-generated repetitions are similar to real repetitions and can increase the insufficiency of workout training data.

4.6 System Implementation and Evaluation

4.6.1 Experimental Setup

mmWave Devices We build a prototype of the proposed system using a single mmWave device, TI AWR1642 [19], which integrates a 2×4 antenna array. The device operates in a frequency range between 77 and 81 GHz. The sampling rate is fixed at 100 frames per second and each frame has 17 chirps. A TI DCA1000EVM [35] data capture card is used to collect data from the mmWave device and send data to a dell laptop for deep model inference.

Fitness Data Collection We recruit 11 volunteers aged from 20 to 44 with various heights from 162 to 185 cm and weights from 50 to 86 kg. The volunteers are asked to perform 14 typical indoor workouts as shown in Table 4.1. The workout data are collected from four different environments (e.g., lounge, corridor, and classroom). We place the mmWave device on a table with a height of 60 cm and the ground truth videos are recorded by a camera. For multi-user scenarios, volunteers are randomly separated into different groups with size from 2 people to 4 people to perform workouts concurrently. During the workouts, all the volunteers are required to keep a reasonable distance from others (e.g., 3 m) to avoid physical touch. During an 8-month survey, we ask each of the volunteers to conduct 20 repetitions for each type of workout. Unless mentioned otherwise, 10 segments are used for training the model, and 10 segments are used to evaluate the performance. In total, we collect over 7000 segments from the volunteers.

Evaluation Metrics To assess the efficacy of our system, we introduce the following evaluation metrics: *Workout Recognition/User Identification Accuracy*, which represents the likelihood that workouts or user identities are accurately

Table 4.1 14 common in-home full-body workouts

W1	Crunches	W8	Squats
W2	Elbow plank and reach	W9	Burpees
W3	Leg raise	W10	High knees
W4	Lunges	W11	Turning kicks
W5	Mountain climber	W12	Chest squeezes
W6	Punches	W13	Side leg raise
W7	Push ups	W14	Side to side chops

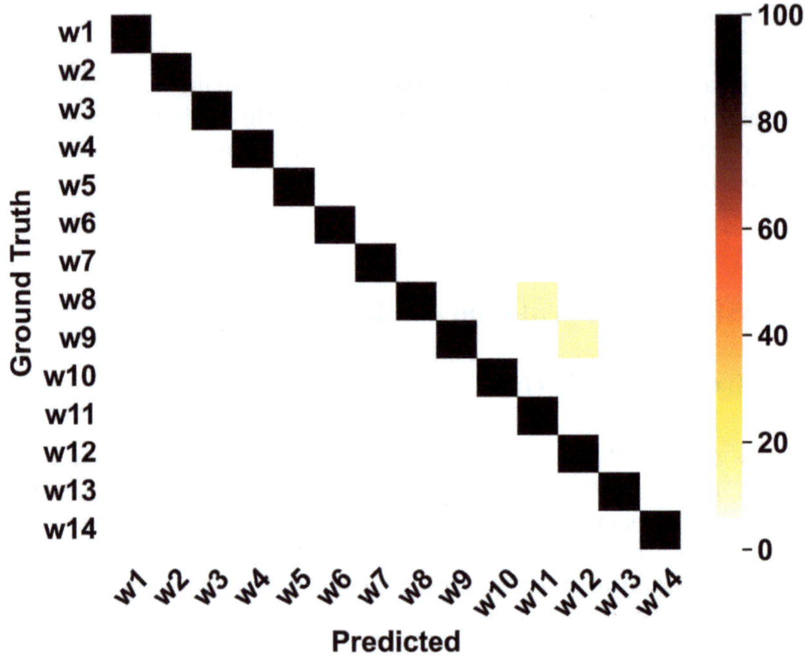

(a)

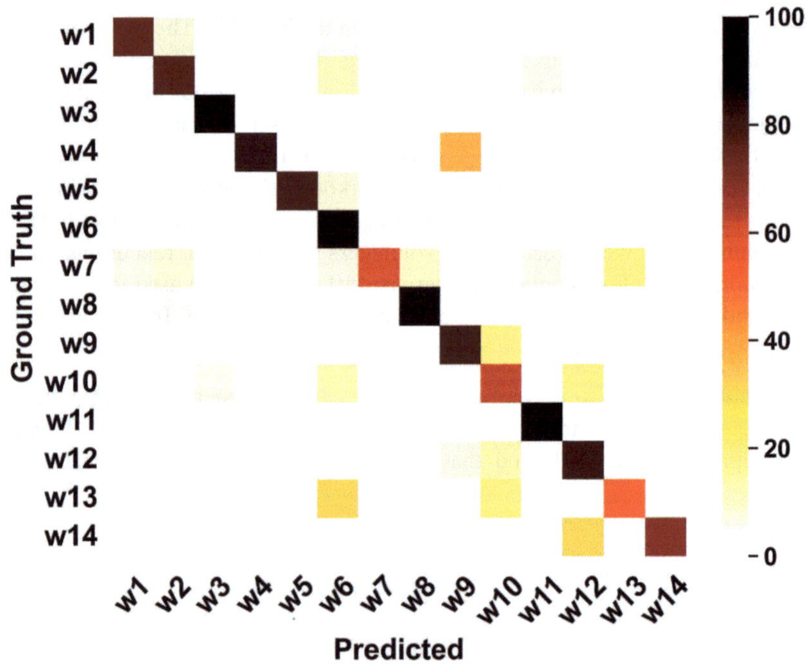

(b)

Fig. 4.9 (**a**) Workout recognition performance of our system with sufficient training data (e.g., 10 repetitions per workout); (**b**) Workout recognition performance without GAN-assisted method when only one real repetition per workout is available; (**c**) Workout recognition performance with GAN-assisted method

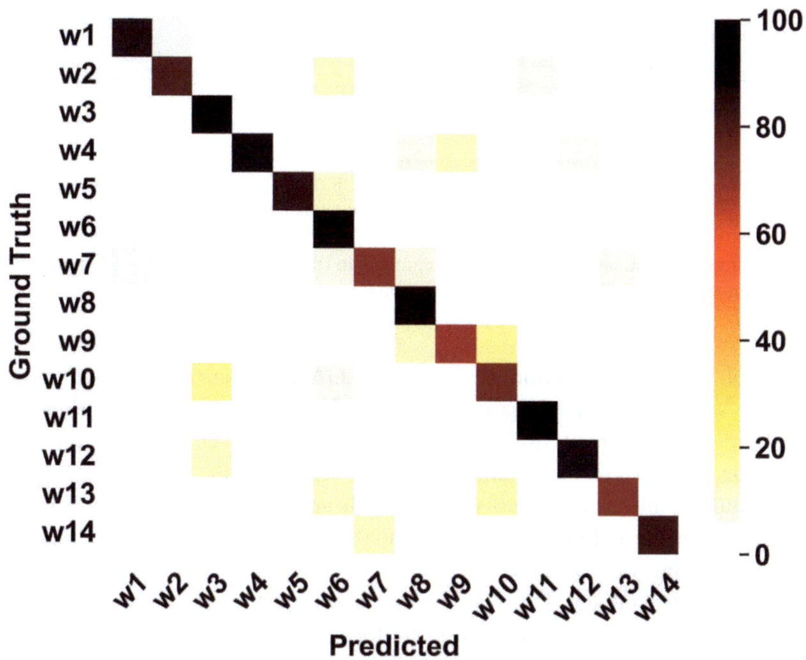

(c)

Fig. 4.9 (continued)

discerned by our system, and the *Confusion Matrix*, which offers a visualization depicting the percentage distribution of each workout identified, encompassing both the accurate workout and alternative possibilities.

4.6.2 Performance of Workout Recognition

We first examine the performance of our system for workout recognition. As demonstrated in Fig. 4.9a, when training data is sufficient (i.e., 10 repetitions per workout per user), our system can achieve an average workout recognition accuracy of 97.69%. Moreover, the recognition accuracy of all workout types is above 87.5%. However, in real-life scenarios, it is usually not practical to ask every user to perform large amounts of workout repetitions of every workout type. For example, when people could only provide a limited amount of repetitions (e.g., one repetition per workout type), a workout recognition system usually could not achieve good performance. In such condition, as shown in Fig. 4.9b, the system's average workout recognition performance is 80%, and the average recognition accuracy for some workout types (i.e., w7, w10, and w13) is even lower than 65%.

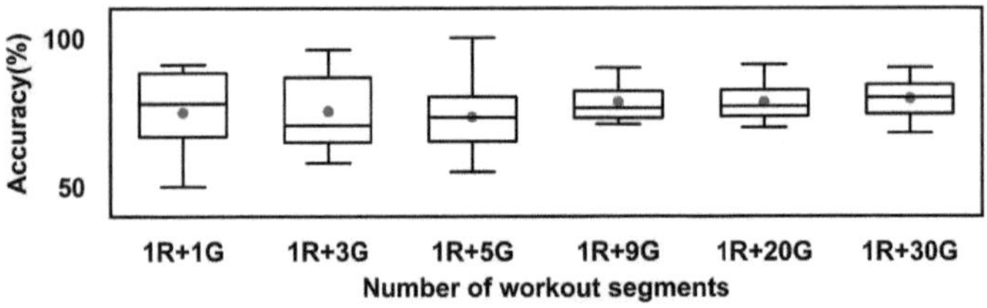

Fig. 4.10 Impact of the number of workout segments in training set (e.g., $1R + 9G$ represents 1 real workout repetition with 9 synthesized repetitions)

To deal with such conditions, we utilize GAN to generate a large number of virtual workout segments based on the limited amount of real workout data and utilize these segments to improve the capability of our system. As shown in Fig. 4.9c, with the GAN-generated workout segments, the workout recognition system could achieve better performance with an average accuracy of 85%. We also notice that the recognition performance for all 14 workouts is increased by at least 3%. Some workouts (w3, w6 and w8) reach a performance of higher than 90% recognition accuracy. This result not only demonstrates that our system could achieve satisfying workout recognition performance with a small amount of real workout training data, but also proves the effectiveness of the proposed GAN-assisted method.

We further explore the minimum number of GAN-generated segments that the system needed to achieve satisfactory performance. Figure 4.10 shows that the average workout recognition accuracy (marked by red points) gradually increases from 74 to 79% when the number of GAN-generated segments of each workout category increases from 1 to 9. However, when more than 9 generated segments are added to the training dataset, the overall accuracy has no obvious further improvement. The result demonstrates that 9 GAN-generated repetitions for each workout/user category is sufficient for our system to achieve obvious performance improvements, thus we use 9 GAN-generated repetitions as our default settings.

4.6.3 *Performance of User Identification*

We then examine the performance of our system for user identification. As is shown in Fig. 4.11a, when training data is sufficient, the user recognition accuracy of all volunteers is higher than 83%. The average accuracy of all users is 92% and the highest accuracy can reach up to 98.33% (U2). We also notice that the performances for some users (e.g., U6) are slightly lower than others, this is because this user has similar body shape and workout patterns with other users. This result shows that our system can identify different users with high accuracy and thus supports personalized workout recognition.

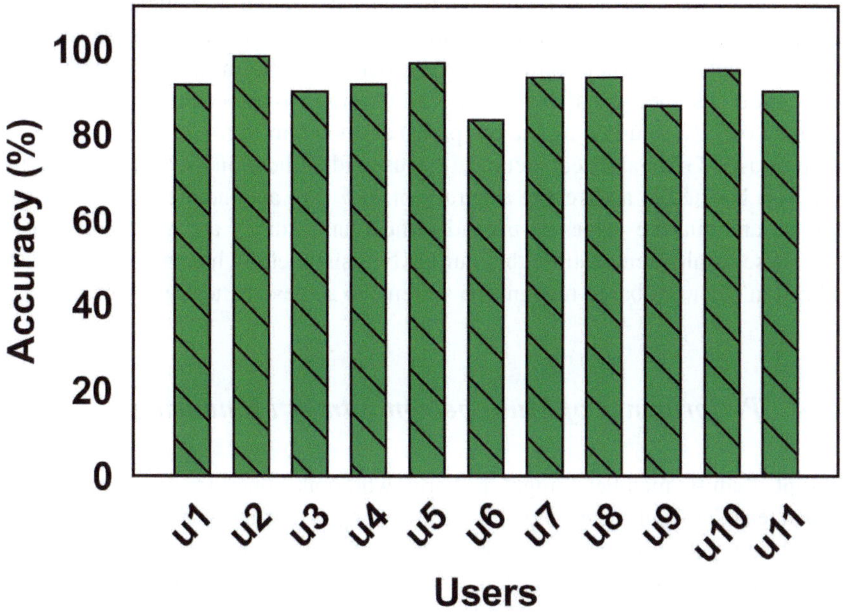

(a)

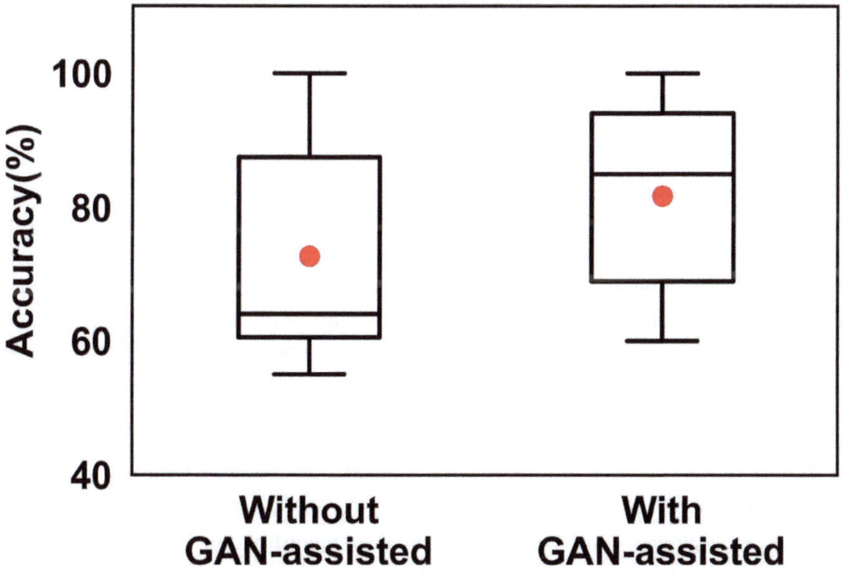

(b)

Fig. 4.11 (**a**) User recognition of our system with sufficient repetition training data (e.g., 10 repetitions per workout); (**b**) User recognition without and with our GAN-assisted method when only one repetition per workout is available

Similar to workout recognition, we further explore the user identification performance of our system when only limited workout data is available. Specifically, we utilize only one repetition per workout per user to train the user classifier. In such conditions, the system only achieves an average user recognition performance accuracy of 72% (marked by the red point) as shown in Fig. 4.11b. However, with the proposed GAN-assisted method, the user identification performance of our system is boosted to an average accuracy of 81%. We also notice that the highest, median, and quartile values of user identification accuracy are all improved over 5%. These results demonstrate that our GAN-assist method has the potential to be utilized in other RF-based recognition systems to achieve better performance.

4.6.4 Performance of Multi-person Fitness Monitoring

Multiple family members might perform workouts concurrently at home. Our system enables multi-user monitoring by using a clustering-based method. To evaluate the performance of our system for multi-user fitness monitoring, we ask multiple people with different group sizes (i.e., 2, 3, and 4) to perform workouts and present the result in Fig. 4.12a. Specifically, in two-user cases, when sufficient training data is available, our system could achieve a workout recognition accuracy of 95% and a user identification accuracy of 90%. When group size increase to three people, our system could achieve a workout recognition accuracy of 90.3% and user identification accuracy of 88.57%. Even when there are four people performing workouts concurrently, our system can still achieve workout recognition accuracy of 85.55% and user identification accuracy of 84%. This result demonstrates that our fitness monitoring system can be applied in family scenarios where generally there will be no more than 4 persons performing workouts together.

Moreover, when family members could only provide a limited amount of repetitions, with the help of our GAN-assisted method, we still observe obvious performance improvements of our system in different scenarios. As shown in Table 4.2, the workout recognition and user identification accuracy in three scenarios have an average improvement of 5.83% and 6.12%, respectively. This result proves that our GAN-assisted method facilitates the practicability of applying our system for family workout monitoring with low training efforts. We further evaluate the impact of distance among users in multi-person scenarios. We ask two volunteers to perform workouts concurrently with a distance of 2, 2.5, and 3 m between each other, respectively. As shown in Fig. 4.12b, our system achieves higher than 90% accuracy in both workout recognition and user identification for all 3 scenarios. Note that the distance among users is selected based on the workout type and the users' heights to avoid touching each other.

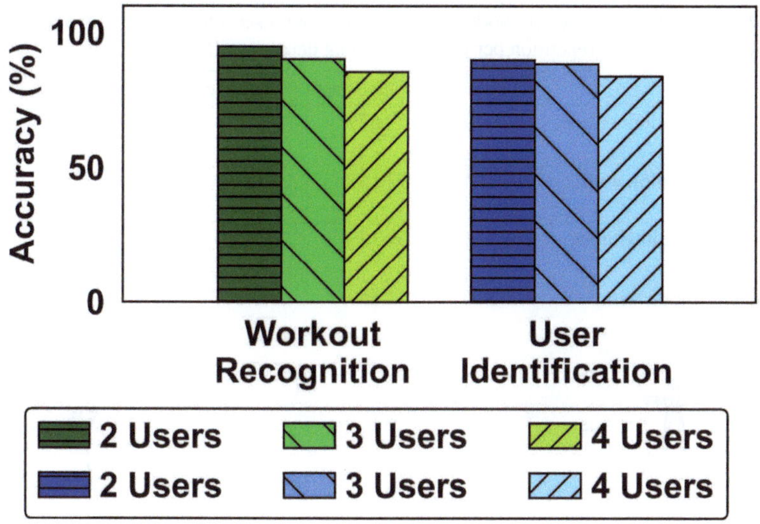

(a)

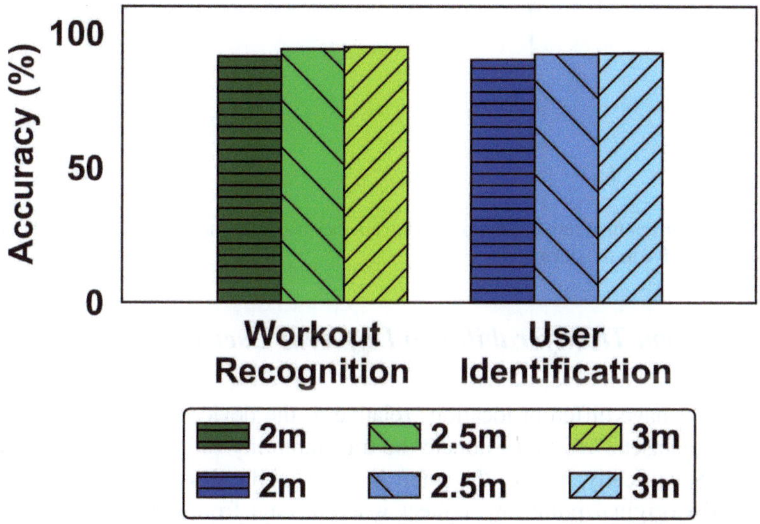

(b)

Fig. 4.12 (**a**) Workout recognition and user identification performance in multi-person scenarios with sufficient training data. (**b**) Impact of distance among users on workout recognition and user identification performance

Table 4.2 The performance of workout recognition and user identification in multi-person scenarios when only one repetition per workout training data is available

	Two users	Three users	Four users	Average improvement
Workout recognition without GAN-assisted	72.73%	69.62%	60.55%	**5.83%**
Workout recognition with GAN-assisted	77.00%	73.15%	70.25%	
User identification without GAN-assisted	69.56%	69.18%	58.25%	**6.12%**
User identification with GAN-assisted	75.93%	71.66%	67.75%	

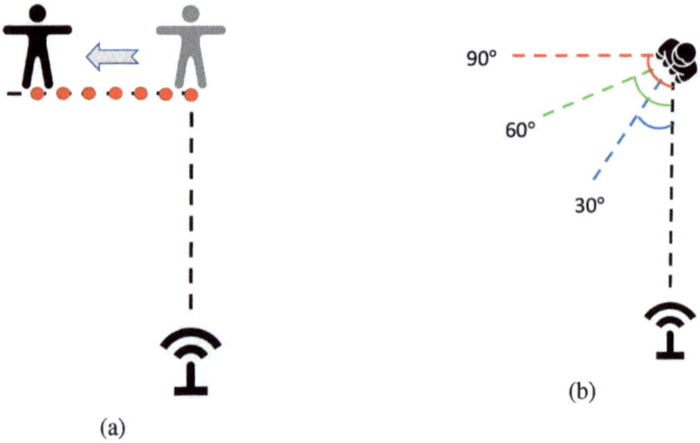

Fig. 4.13 (**a**) Different relative locations between the user and the device; (**b**) Different face orientations relative to the device

4.6.5 System Transferability to Different User Locations

People might have different locations relative to the devices between the training and testing datasets. We first evaluate the transferability of our system to different locations. Specifically, we set the point in front of the device with a distance of 2.5 m as the original point. We collect workout data from 6 new locations (i.e., each has a distance ranging from 15 to 90 cm to the original point) with an interval of 15 cm as shown in Fig. 4.13a. We use workouts collected at original point as the source domain and all the workouts collected at other locations as the target domain. In addition, to evaluate the transferability of our system to users' different face orientations, we also set the direction that faces the device as the original orientation. The volunteers are asked to perform workouts at the same location with 7 different face orientations (i.e., 0° to 90° with an interval of 15°) as shown in Fig. 4.13b. Workouts collected at 0° are used as the source domain while workouts collected at other orientations are chosen as the target domain.

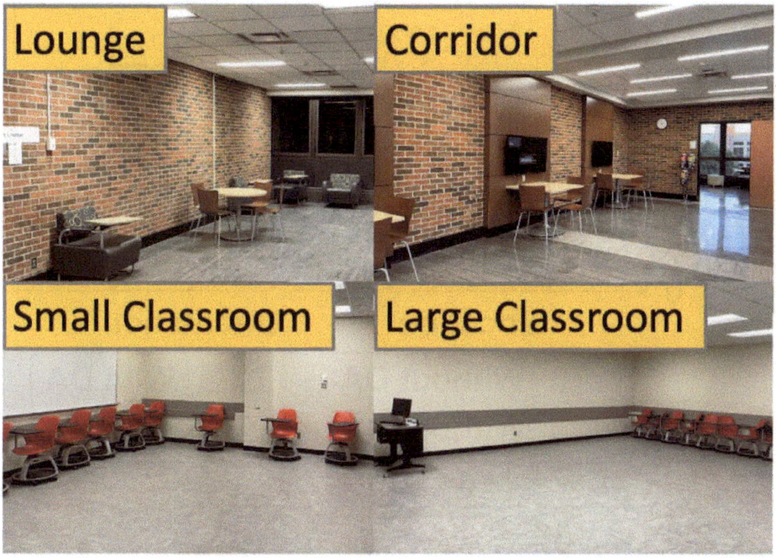

Fig. 4.14 Different environments between the training and testing datasets

We evaluate the performance of our system via training the deep learning model with workouts collected from the source domain and adapt the model to the target domain using the domain adaptation framework. For comparison, we also examined the deep learning model without domain adaptation. As shown in Fig. 4.15a, we observe that without domain adaptation, the performance of workout recognition is low (i.e., 75.25% across different locations and 61.37% across various orientations). Our domain adaptation framework boosts the system's workout recognition performance on new locations and orientations to 89.5 and 84.45%, respectively. The result demonstrates that the proposed domain adaptation method can alleviate the impact of different locations/orientations between training and testing data on our system.

4.6.6 System Transferability to Different Environments

To evaluate the transferability of our system to different environments, we collect workout data from 4 different rooms with various furniture layouts: a lounge with a size of $7 \times 4\,\text{m}^2$, a corridor with a size of $10 \times 4\,\text{m}^2$, and two classrooms with the size of $6 \times 8\,\text{m}^2$ and $10 \times 10\,\text{m}^2$, respectively, as shown in Fig. 4.14. In each environment, the data are collected with the same location and face orientation relative to the device. Workouts collected in one environment is chosen as the source domain while workouts collected in another environment is selected as the target domain. We test all 6 source-target evaluation pairs and present the result in Fig. 4.15b. We

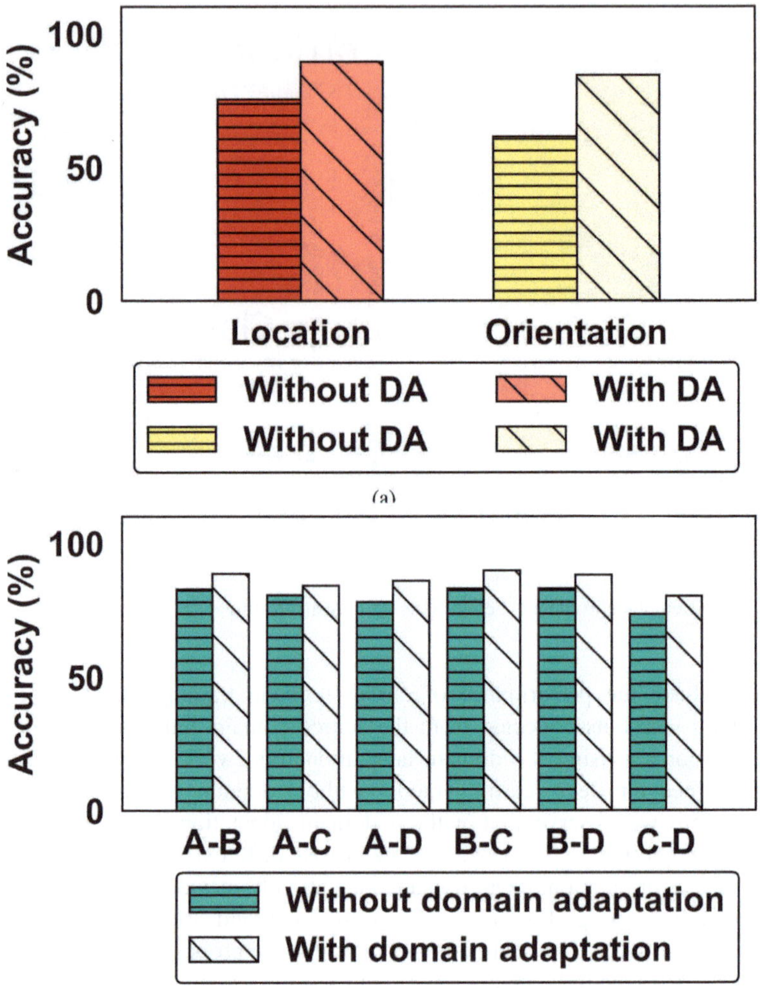

(b)

Fig. 4.15 (**a**) Workout recognition without and with domain adaptation (DA) across different relative locations and face orientations; (**b**) Workout recognition without and with domain adaptation across different environments (e.g., A–B represents training data from Environment A and testing data from Environment B)

observe that with the help of domain adaptation framework, our system achieves 86% workout recognition accuracy with an average 4% improvement compared with not using domain adaptation. We also note that our system still achieves good transferability across different environments even without using domain adaptation training which validates the effectiveness of our environmental impact mitigation methods. The above results show that our system can be easily deployed across different room environments. This type of flexibility is essential to the practical fitness system deployment in everyday life.

4.7 Summary

In this chapter, we present a novel multi-person fitness monitoring system that utilizes a single Commercial Off-The-Shelf (COTS) mmWave device. Our system seamlessly integrates several essential modules, including workout recognition, user identification, multi-user monitoring, and training effort reduction, into a unified framework. To address the issue of extensive training requirements, we have devised a domain adaptation framework that effectively reduces the need for collecting large volumes of training data from various domains. By mitigating the impact of domain-specific characteristics embedded in mmWave signals, our framework minimizes the data collection efforts. Furthermore, we have developed a GAN-assisted method to enhance user identification and workout recognition even when the availability of training data from the same domain is limited. To achieve personalized workout recognition, we propose a novel spatial-temporal heatmap feature that seamlessly integrates multiple workout characteristics. Additionally, we have devised a clustering-based approach for concurrent workout monitoring, enabling efficient tracking and analysis of multiple workouts. Through rigorous experimentation involving 14 typical workouts with the participation of 11 individuals, we have demonstrated the effectiveness of our system. Remarkably, our system achieves an impressive accuracy of 85% and 81% for workout recognition and user identification, respectively, by utilizing just one sample of each workout and user.

References

1. Akpa, E.A.H., Fujiwara, M., Arakawa, Y., Suwa, H., Yasumoto, K.: Gift: Glove for indoor fitness tracking system. In: 2018 IEEE International Conference on Pervasive Computing and Communications Workshops (PerCom Workshops) (2018). https://doi.org/10.1109/PERCOMW.2018.8480211
2. Alam, M.A.U., Rahman, M.M., Widberg, J.Q.: Palmar: Towards adaptive multi-inhabitant activity recognition in point-cloud technology. Preprint (2021). arXiv:2106.11902
3. Celiktutan, O., Akgul, C.B., Wolf, C., Sankur, B.: Graph-based analysis of physical exercise actions. In: Proceedings of the 1st ACM International Workshop on Multimedia Indexing and Information Retrieval for Healthcare, MIIRH '13. Association for Computing Machinery, New York (2013). https://doi.org/10.1145/2505323.2505330
4. Dummies: Weight training: How many reps (and sets) to do (2019). https://www.dummies.com/health/exercise/weights/weight-training-how-many-reps-and-sets-to-do/
5. Frid-Adar, M., Klang, E., Amitai, M., Goldberger, J., Greenspan, H.: Synthetic data augmentation using gan for improved liver lesion classification (2018). https://doi.org/10.1109/ISBI.2018.8363576

6. Ganin, Y., Ustinova, E., Ajakan, H., Germain, P., Larochelle, H., Laviolette, F., Marchand, M., Lempitsky, V.: Domain-adversarial training of neural networks. J. Mach. Learn. Res. **17**, 1–35 (2016)
7. Ghorbel, E., Boutteau, R., Boonaert, J., Savatier, X., Lecoeuche, S.: Kinematic spline curves: a temporal invariant descriptor for fast action recognition. Image Vision Comput. **77**, 60–71 (2018)
8. Guo, X., Liu, J., Shi, C., Liu, H., Chen, Y., Chuah, M.C.: Device-free personalized fitness assistant using wifi. In: Proceedings of the ACM on Interactive, Mobile, Wearable and Ubiquitous Technologies (2018)
9. Hassana, M.M., Uddin, Z., Mohamed, A., Almogrena, A.: A robust human activity recognition system using smartphone sensors and deep learning. Future Gener. Comput. Syst. **81**, 307–313 (2018)
10. Jiang, W., Miao, C., Ma, F., Yao, S., Wang, Y., Yuan, Y., Xue, H., Song, C., Ma, X., Koutsonikolas, D., Xu, W., Su, L.: Towards environment independent device free human activity recognition. In: Proceedings of the 24th Annual International Conference on Mobile Computing and Networking, MobiCom '18. Association for Computing Machinery, New York (2018). https://doi.org/10.1145/3241539.3241548
11. Jin, F., Zhang, R., Sengupta, A., Cao, S., Hariri, S., Agarwal, N.K., Agarwal, S.K.: Multiple patients behavior detection in real-time using mmwave radar and deep cnns. In: 2019 IEEE Radar Conference (RadarConf). IEEE (2019)
12. Jin, F., Sengupta, A., Cao, S.: mmfall: Fall detection using 4-d mmwave radar and a hybrid variational rnn autoencoder. IEEE Trans. Autom. Sci. Eng. **19**(2), 1245–1257 (2020)
13. Langford-Smith, F., et al.: Radiotron Designer's Handbook. Wireless Press, Sydney (1941)
14. Liu, H., Wang, Y., Zhou, A., He, H., Wang, W., Wang, K., Pan, P., Lu, Y., Liu, L., Ma, H.: Real-time arm gesture recognition in smart home scenarios via millimeter wave sensing. In: Proceedings of the ACM on Interactive, Mobile, Wearable and Ubiquitous Technologies (2020)
15. van der Maaten, L., Hinton, G.: Visualizing data using t-sne. J. Mach. Learn. Res. (2008). http://jmlr.org/papers/v9/vandermaaten08a.html
16. Meng, Y., Yi, S.H., Kim, H.C.: Health and wellness monitoring using intelligent sensing technique. J. Indian Prosthodont. Soc. **15**(3), 478–491 (2019)
17. Moradi, M., Madani, A., Karargyris, A., Syeda-Mahmood, T.: Chest x-ray generation and data augmentation for cardiovascular abnormality classification (2018). https://doi.org/10.1117/12.2293971
18. Pegoraro, J., Meneghello, F., Rossi, M.: Multiperson continuous tracking and identification from mm-wave micro-doppler signatures. IEEE Trans. Geosci. Remote Sensing **59**(4), 2994–3009 (2020)
19. Pirkani, A.A., Pooni, S., Cherniakov, M.: Implementation of mimo beamforming on an ots fmcw automotive radar (2019). https://doi.org/10.23919/IRS.2019.8768103
20. Qian, X., Fu, Y., Xiang, T., Wang, W., Qiu, J., Wu, Y., Jiang, Y.G., Xue, X.: Pose-normalized image generation for person re-identification. In: Proceedings of the European Conference on Computer Vision (2018)
21. Radartutorial: Frequency-modulated continuous-wave radar (fmcw radar) (1998). https://www.radartutorial.eu
22. Ren, Y., Lu, J., Beletchi, A., Huang, Y., Karmanov, I., Fontijne, D., Patel, C., Xu, H.: Hand gesture recognition using 802.11 ad mmwave sensor in the mobile device. In: 2021 IEEE Wireless Communications and Networking Conference Workshops (WCNCW). IEEE (2021)
23. Santhalingam, P.S., Hosain, A.A., Zhang, D., Pathak, P., Rangwala, H., Kushalnagar, R.: mmasl: Environment-independent asl gesture recognition using 60 ghz millimeter-wave signals. In: Proceedings of ACM on Interactive, Mobile, Wearable and Ubiquitous Technologies (2020)
24. Sengupta, A., Jin, F., Zhang, R., Cao, S.: mm-pose: real-time human skeletal posture estimation using mmwave radars and cnns. IEEE Sensors J. **20**, 10032–10044 (2020)

25. Su, C.J., Chiang, C.Y., Huang, J.Y.: Kinect-enabled home-based rehabilitation system using dynamic time warping and fuzzy logic. Appl. Soft Comput. (2014). https://doi.org/10.1016/j.asoc.2014.04.020. https://www.sciencedirect.com/science/article/pii/S1568494614001859
26. Tiwari, G., Gupta, S.: An mmwave radar based real-time contactless fitness tracker using deep cnns. IEEE Sensors J. **21**, 17262–17270 (2021)
27. Wang, Y., Liu, J., Chen, Y., Gruteser, M., Yang, J., Liu, H.: E-eyes: Device-free location-oriented activity identification using fine-grained wifi signatures. In: Proceedings of the 20th Annual International Conference on Mobile Computing and Networking, MobiCom '14. Association for Computing Machinery, New York (2014). https://doi.org/10.1145/2639108.2639143
28. Wang, J., Zhang, L., Wang, C., Ma, X., Gao, Q., Lin, B.: Device-free human gesture recognition with generative adversarial networks. IEEE Internet Things J. **7**, 7678–7688 (2020)
29. Wang, Y., Liu, H., Cui, K., Zhou, A., Li, W., Ma, H.: m-activity: Accurate and real-time human activity recognition via millimeter wave radar. In: ICASSP 2021–2021 IEEE International Conference on Acoustics, Speech and Signal Processing (ICASSP). IEEE (2021)
30. Wu, C., Zhang, F., Wang, B., Liu, K.R.: mmtrack: Passive multi-person localization using commodity millimeter wave radio. In: IEEE INFOCOM 2020. IEEE (2020)
31. Xue, H., Ju, Y., Miao, C., Wang, Y., Wang, S., Zhang, A., Su, L.: mmmesh: Towards 3d real-time dynamic human mesh construction using millimeter-wave. In: Proceedings of the 19th Annual International Conference on Mobile Systems, Applications, and Services (2021)
32. Zhao, M., Li, T., Abu Alsheikh, M., Tian, Y., Zhao, H., Torralba, A., Katabi, D.: Through-wall human pose estimation using radio signals. In: Proceedings of the IEEE Conference on Computer Vision and Pattern Recognition (2018)
33. Zhao, M., Tian, Y., Zhao, H., Alsheikh, M.A., Li, T., Hristov, R., Kabelac, Z., Katabi, D., Torralba, A.: Rf-based 3d skeletons. In: Proceedings of the 2018 Conference of the ACM Special Interest Group on Data Communication (2018)
34. Zhao, M., Liu, Y., Raghu, A., Li, T., Zhao, H., Torralba, A., Katabi, D.: Through-wall human mesh recovery using radio signals. In: Proceedings of the IEEE International Conference on Computer Vision (2019)
35. Zhenyu, L.Z., Lu, W., Wu, J., Yang, S., Li, G.: A pelt-kcn algorithm for fmcw radar interference suppression based on signal reconstruction. IEEE Access (2020). https://doi.org/10.1109/ACCESS.2020.2977098

Chapter 5
Non-intrusive Eating Habits Monitoring Using Millimeter Wave

The potential applications of mmWave technologies are vast and diverse. In this chapter, we aim to explore the feasibility of harnessing millimeter wave technology as an unobtrusive method for eating habits monitoring. The significance of maintaining good health is intrinsically linked to dietary habits. An unhealthy diet can be a precursor to an array of health complications such as obesity, diabetes, heart diseases, and an increased risk of cancers, etc. To aid individuals in keeping track of their dietary behaviors, it is crucial to implement an effective monitoring system. However, conventional sensor-based and camera-based dietary monitoring systems have limitations. They either require users to wear specialized devices, or might raise privacy concerns. Similarly, while WiFi-based methods have demonstrated reasonable performance in specific cases, they have their own set of constraints. Wireless signals often carry environment-specific information, thereby impacting the accuracy of monitoring eating activities. To overcome these challenges, we propose to implement a millimeter wave-enabled eating behavior monitoring system that operates independently of any environment. Our system introduces an innovative approach that mitigates the influence of the surroundings by analyzing mmWave signals in the Doppler-Range domain. This allows us to achieve meticulous monitoring of eating behaviors, facilitated by the construction of a Spatial-Temporal Heatmap through the integration of multiple measurements. Consequently, we can differentiate between dietary activities performed with various utensils such as forks, knives, spoons, chopsticks, or even bare hands. Moreover, we leverage unsupervised learning-based 2D segmentation and an eating period derivation algorithm to accurately estimate the duration of each eating activity. Additionally, our system showcases the potential to infer food categories and determine eating speed. Extensive experiments involving over 1000 eating activities demonstrate the effectiveness of our system, achieving high accuracy in dietary activity recognition with a low false detection rate.

The reminder of this chapter is organized as follows. We present the research background in Sect. 5.1, followed by a review of existing work in Sect. 5.2. In

X. Guo et al., *Mobile Technologies for Smart Healthcare System Design*,
Wireless Networks, https://doi.org/10.1007/978-3-031-57345-3_5

Sect. 5.3, we discuss the system design for non-intrusive eating habits derivation using millimeter wave. Subsequently, Sect. 5.4 provides detailed information on environment-invariant eating monitoring. The system implementation and evaluation will be covered in Sect. 5.5. Finally, we conclude the chapter with a summary in Sect. 5.6.

5.1 Background

Dietary is an important activity in people's daily lives since it is closely related to individuals' health conditions. Centers for Disease Control and Prevention (CDC) shows that an unhealthy diet can cause obesity, diabetes, heart diseases, as well as increase the risk of over 13 types of cancers [2]. A recent study [3] has shown that unhealthy diet contributes to approximately 678,000 deaths each year in the U.S. Thus, it is necessary to develop a monitoring system that can help individuals keep tracking their dietary behaviors and offer them useful suggestions.

Eating behavior monitoring can provide essential information (e.g., food categories, eating speed) for dietary behavior analysis and provide useful recommendations if poor dietary behaviors are detected. Traditional eating monitoring systems [4, 7] use cameras to take images or videos of users to track their dietary information. However, those vision-based methods may raise potential privacy concerns from collecting images or videos of users. In contrast, recent studies [1, 13] propose to use wearable sensors for dietary monitoring. Though sensor-based methods do not raise privacy concerns, they require users to wear one or multiple sensors during eating. Therefore, this kind of methods is not only inconvenient but also impractical.

All the aforementioned shortcomings of existing systems contribute to the emergence of device-free monitoring systems such as WiFi-based methods. Lin et al. propose WiEat [5], which utilizes channel state information extracted from WiFi devices to recognize different dietary activities. However, as WiFi signals are sensitive to surrounding environments and are vulnerable to interference, more stable and stronger signals are desired for eating monitoring tasks. Recent years have witnessed the success of using mmWave signals for posture estimation [8] or activity recognition [9]. This is because mmWave signals have more stable and higher-resolution with shorter wavelengths and stronger directivity. In this chapter, we propose to design an eating behavior monitoring system via mmWave techniques which have already been integrated into the new generation WiFi standards (i.e., IEEE 802.11ad).

In order to utilize mmWave signals for eating behavior monitoring, several challenges should be addressed in practice. First, people usually eat in different places (e.g., dining room, living room) every day. Traditional WiFi-based eating monitoring systems that are trained in a specific environment will typically not work well when being applied in a different environment. To solve this problem, in this work, we propose an environmental impact mitigation method by subtracting the static component from every frame in the Dopper-Range domain. Our eating monitoring system is environment-invariant and can be applied to new environments without extra training. Moreover, in the real world, people might perform non-eating activities throughout the day. Hence, we develop a dietary activity detection method to detect eating activities automatically based on the repetitive velocity pattern of eating activity in the time domain. Furthermore, fine-grained eating behavior monitoring requires differentiation among eating activities with various utensils (e.g, eating with a fork or spoon). However, different dietary activities are hard to be distinguished since they all involve hand movements with similar ranges. To address this problem, we construct Spatial-Temporal Heatmap by integrating velocity information from every distance measurement in the Doppler-Range domain and combining them with time information. Besides, we utilize an unsupervised learning-based 2D segmentation algorithm to facilitate accurate dietary activity recognition. We further develop a deep neural network to extract the unique characteristics of every eating activity and classify them based on the utensils used (i.e., fork, fork&knife, spoon, chopsticks, bare hand). In addition, to further derive detailed dietary behavior information, we estimate the eating period of every eating activity and infer the eating duration and speed of meals.

The contributions of this chapter are summarized as follows. As far as we know, our system is the first eating behavior monitoring system using a COTS mmWave radar sensor. Our proposed system constructs unique environment-invariant Spatial-Temporal signal representations that integrate velocity, time duration, and range of movement information. It has the capability of eliminating environmental impact from static objects and differentiating eating activities from daily activities. Additionally, we develop a fine-tuned deep neural network to facilitate accurate dietary activity recognition. Extensive experiments involving six individuals and over 1000 eating activities demonstrate that our system achieves dietary activity recognition with an average accuracy of 97.5% and a false detection rate of 5%.

5.2 Related Work

Traditional eating monitoring systems widely use Vision-based methods [4, 7]. Such methods use cameras to take images or videos when users eat meals for further analysis. DietCam [4] exploits photos or videos taken by commercial mobile devices to perform dietary monitoring. Another system developed by O'Loughlin et al. [7] exploits Microsoft SenseCams to capture videos and estimate the dietary energy intake. Such vision-based methods usually raise potential privacy concerns since the camera may capture users' private information such as social relationships and location privacy.

Some existing work tend to use wearable sensors for dietary monitoring to avoid potential privacy concerns in vision-based methods. Amft et al. [1] use a condenser microphone to detect air-conducted vibrations caused by chewing to determine food textures. Zhang et al. [13] propose an accelerometer-based wearable device attached to users' wrists to detect eating activities based on the three-dimensional kinematics movement model. Though sensor-based methods may not have privacy concerns, users are required to wear one or multiple sensors during eating. Therefore, they are both inconvenient and impractical.

Recently, radio frequency (RF) signals have been proposed to address the above limitations. As a prevalent RF sensing modality, WiFi signals have shown initial success in many activity recognition applications. Wang et al. develop E-eyes [12], which exploits WiFi signals to provide device-free human activity identification. Lin et al. develop WiEat [5] that can achieve high accuracy in device-free dietary monitoring using commercial WiFi devices. However, WiFi-based methods are sensitive to environmental changes. Millimeter wave (mmWave) has been proven more robust than WiFi due to its high bandwidth and native beam-forming technology. Existing mmWave-based systems like [8] and [9] often focus on posture estimation or activity recognition. None of them show that their system can distinguish eating activities with minute differences in hand or finger movements and provide fine-grained analysis of eating activities. This chapter develops a system leveraging mmWave signals from commodity mmWave devices to provide fine-grained dietary monitoring.

5.3 Non-intrusive Eating Habits Monitoring System Design

The goal of our system is to provide environment-invariant fine-grained eating behavior monitoring by leveraging a single commercial mmWave device. Toward this end, we develop a low-cost mmWave-based eating behavior monitoring system. The system takes as input the mmWave signals reflected from the human body. The system first performs signal processing to derive the velocity, distance information of the user's activity from the received mmWave signals. Then, it eliminates the impact from environment by subtracting signals reflected off static objects. Next, we construct Spatial-Temporal Heatmap to aggregate the instantaneous velocity from every distance measurement in the Doppler-Range domain and combine them with time information. Such integrated multidimensional signal representation can facilitate fine-grained activity recognition. We propose a dietary activity detection method based on the repetitive eating activity patterns in the time domain to detect dietary activities based on the Spatial-Temporal signal representation. To further differentiate eating activities, we apply DBSCAN [10] to cluster and segment each activity, and develop a deep neural network to identify them. The last component of our proposed system is eating period monitoring which estimates the eating period of each eating activity. Such information is useful to assist various health-related problems, such as diabetes, heart diseases, etc. The overview of the proposed system is shown in Fig. 5.1.

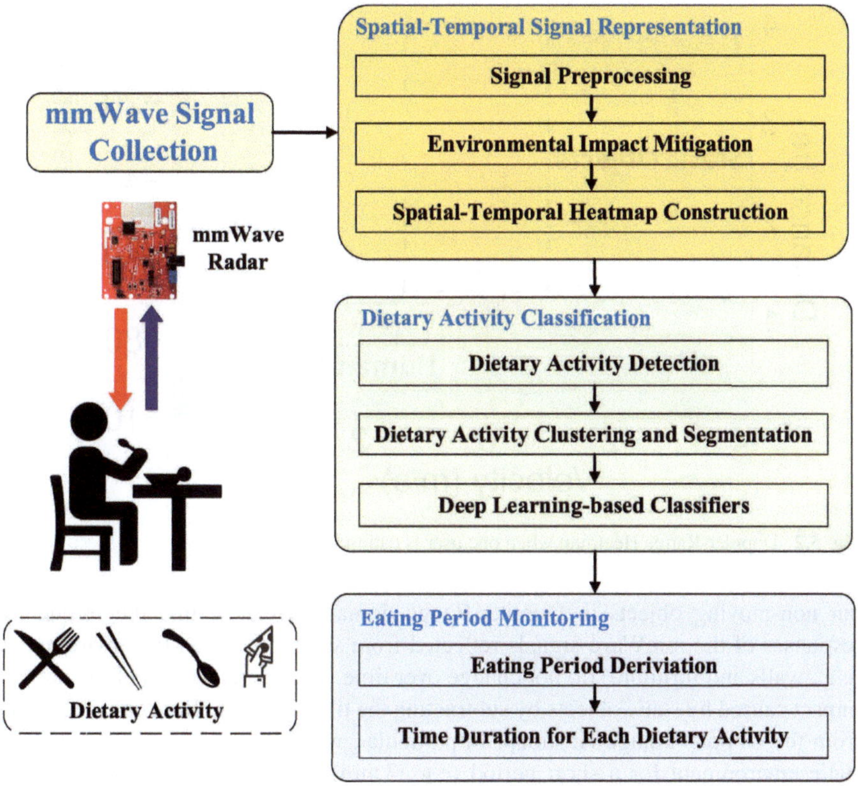

Fig. 5.1 System overview of eating habits derivation using millimeter wave

5.4 Environment-invariant Eating Monitoring

5.4.1 Spatial-temporal Signal Representation and Heatmap Construction

Signal Preprocessing We first perform range-FFT and Doppler-FFT on the received mmWave signals to derive the distance and velocity information of a user's activity respectively. Then, we derive the Doppler-Range Heatmap based on the instant velocity and distance measurements. As shown in Fig. 5.2, the heatmap indicates the strength of frequency responses of the reflected signals via the color. However, since static objects (e.g., furniture and walls) in the environments can also reflect mmWave signals, it is still hard to extract signals from the human in the Doppler-Range Heatmap.

Environmental Impact Mitigation To eliminate the environmental impact mentioned above, we propose an environmental impact mitigation method by filtering

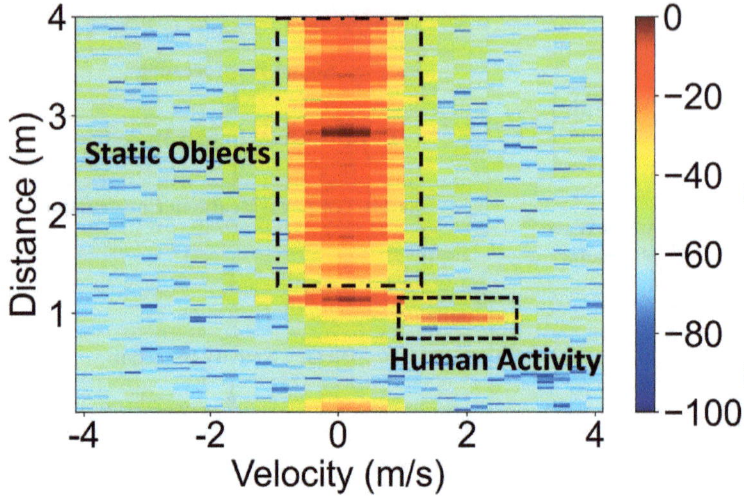

Fig. 5.2 Doppler-Range Heatmap when one user is eating using a fork

out non-moving objects in Doppler-Range domain. We note that the frequency responses of the mmWave signals reflected from static objects in the environment (e.g., walls and furniture) do not change over time. Therefore, we can eliminate the impact caused by static objects by subtracting the time-invariant frequency response from the Doppler-Range Heatmap. In particular, we collect mmWave signals in a static environment for a short period (e.g., 3 min) and derive the Doppler-Range Heatmap to estimate the time-invariant frequency response.

Spatial-Temporal Heatmap Construction Although the denoised Doppler-Range Heatmap can capture the instant velocities at different distances, it is not enough to describe the process of the dietary activities. We propose a more comprehensive signal representation by constructing the Spatial-Temporal Heatmap that contains the temporal information of eating activities (e.g., time duration of each activity and variation of velocity with time). Specifically, we accumulate the velocity measurements of each distance in every Doppler-Range Heatmap frame and then present their dynamics in the time domain as follows:

$$V_{q,t} = \sum_{p=1}^{D} (f_{p,q,t}) \times v_{p,t}, \; p \in [1, D], q \in [1, R], \tag{5.1}$$

where $f_{p,q,t}$ is the strength of a frequency response in the Doppler-Range Heatmap, p is the doppler index, q is the range index, t is the frame index, and $v_{p,t}$ is the velocity corresponding to a Doppler index p at frame t. Then we normalize the derived $V_{q,t}$ to $[-1, 1]$ and map the original 2-dimensional Doppler-Range data to a more comprehensive 3-dimensional Spacial-Temporal Heatmap, which presents the process of the eating activities as shown in Fig. 5.3.

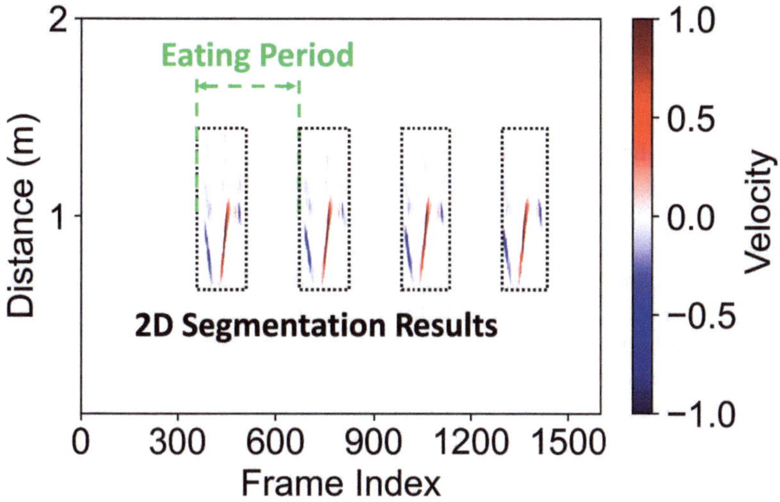

Fig. 5.3 Spatial-Temporal Heatmap of four eating activities using a fork

5.4.2 Dietary Activity Detection and Classification

Dietary Activity Detection After constructing Spatial-Temporal signal representations from mmWave signals, we perform the dietary activity detection to determine whether the mmWave signals contain dietary activities or not. We find that dietary activities usually have repetitive patterns in the Spatial-Temporal domain while non-dietary activities do not. The reason for this observation is that dietary activities consist of repetitive hand and arm movements that bring food to the mouth from the table. As a result, we propose to detect dietary activities by searching the repetitive patterns in the Spatial-Temporal Heatmap using a sliding window. Particularly, we accumulate the velocities from all the distances at a particular time in a frame to transfer the heatmap to one-dimensional data. We use an autocorrelation-based method to determine whether the mmWave signals contain a repetitive pattern or not. We empirically determine that a dietary activity is detected when the number of peaks in the autocorrelation results is more than five.

Dietary Activity Clustering and 2D Segmentation Once a dietary activity is detected, the system performs the dietary activity segmentation to focus on the signals related to dietary activities. The basic idea is to determine each dietary activity's time duration and range of movement in the Spatial-Temporal Heatmap. We first remove the points with low absolute velocity from the heatmap based on an empirical threshold. Then, we utilize an unsupervised learning-based clustering method (i.e., DBSCAN) to separate the points into different clusters. We design a dynamic algorithm to determine the 2D window size of each activity based on its time duration and range of movement. Particularly, for each cluster, we determine the window size based on the differences between the coordinates of the edge points in the Spatial-Temporal plane. The box in Fig. 5.3 illustrates the 2D segmentation results of our algorithm. In addition, we scale up the size of the window by an empirical constant (i.e., 1.2) to ensure that it contains all the signals related to dietary activities.

Deep Learning-based Classifier Design We choose to use neural network-based method for final classification since it has shown robust performance in image classification tasks [11]. The segments derived by the proposed segmentation method are first resized to images with size of 224 × 224. Our convolutional neural network contains nine layers. Three convolutional layers are exploited for up-sampling, three Max Pooling layers with each follows a convolutional layer are used for down-sampling. After the process of three rounds of up-sampling and down-sampling, a 64-dimensional feature map is obtained and a flatten layer is followed to reduce the feature map into a one-dimension array. Two dense layers at the end of the network will classify arrays into five categories, each category is mapped to a specific dietary activity.

5.4.3 Eating Period Monitoring

Researchers [6] have demonstrated that the speed of eating is an important factor for weight control. People eating quickly have a significantly higher possibility to develop obesity. The basic idea of eating period monitoring is to derive the accurate time duration of each eating activity and infer detailed eating information (e.g., eating period of a meal, eating speed). Given this objective, we propose an eating period derivation method. We infer the time duration of each eating activity based on calculating the interval with neighboring activities. Specifically, as shown in Fig. 5.3, we determine the beginning of each eating activity by searching the time stamp of the left edge from the 2D segmentation box. We then estimate the eating period of each eating activity based on the differences between consecutive time stamps. By estimating the time duration of each eating activity, we could further infer the accumulated eating period using specific utensils during a meal, which could be used to estimate other high-level information such as the calorie intake and nutrition balance. In addition, the number of eating activities during a meal and average eating period could also be used to detect poor dietary behaviors of users, such as overeating and eating too quickly.

5.5 System Implementation and Evaluation

5.5.1 Experimental Setup

mmWave Devices In our experiments, we use a single TI AWR1642 commercial mmWave radar equipped with a 2 × 4 antenna array. The radar operates at a

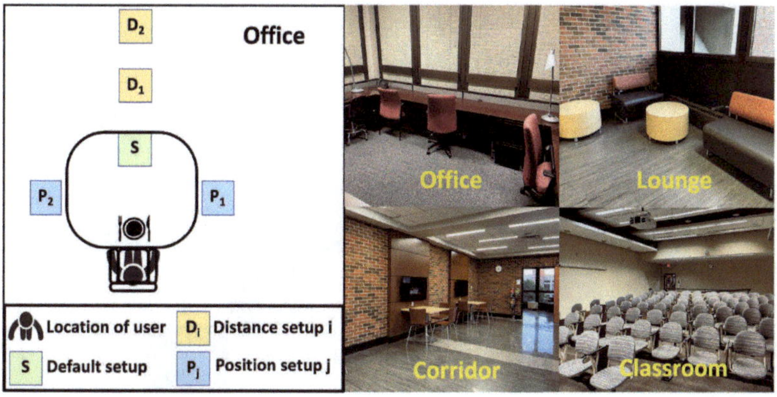

Fig. 5.4 Experiment setup

frequency band between 77 and 81 GHz with a sampling rate fixed at 100 frames per second. All devices are attached to a DELL G3 laptop for deep learning model inference.

Data Collection We conduct our experiments by recruiting 6 volunteers (age from 22 to 40). The profiles are collected at an office with a size of 5×3 m^2. A total of five typical eating activities are performed by the volunteers. Over 1000 eating activity data are collected and the ground truths are measured and verified by camera-based method during the experiments. As is shown in Fig. 5.4, we totally test three different positions and three distances (1, 1.5 and 2 m) to evaluate impact of device positions and distances. For the evaluation of environment impact, we collect data under three different environments: (a). a lounge with a size of 4×4 m^2; (b). a corridor with a size of 5×9 m^2; (c). a classroom with a size of 9×15 m^2.

Evaluation Metrics We define four different evaluation metrics: *Dietary Activity Recognition Accuracy* which is the percentage of predicted dietary activities that are correctly recognized among all activities, *False Detection Rate (FDR)* defined as the ratio between the number of incorrectly classified activities and the total number of activities, *Confusion Matrix* presenting the percentage of a specific activity being identified among all the activities, and *Estimated Error* defining the difference between the estimated eating duration and actual eating duration for a single dietary activity.

5.5.2 Performance of Dietary Activity Classification

In this section, we first compare the overall performance of the proposed CNN-based classification method with traditional classifiers. Figure 5.5 demonstrates the

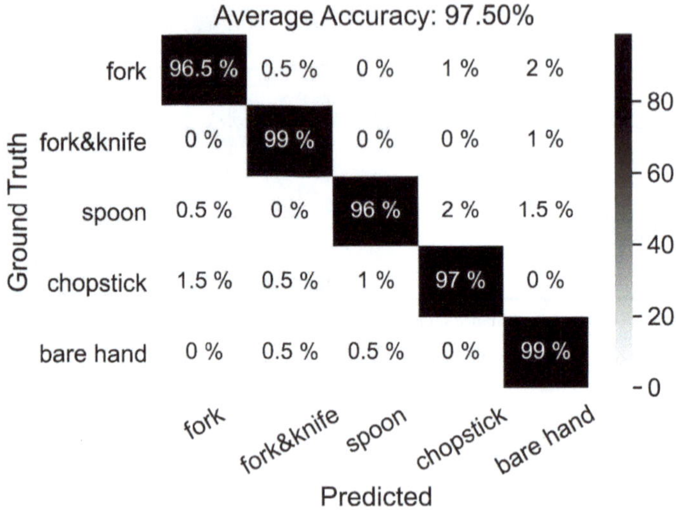

Fig. 5.5 Confusion matrix of dietary activity classification using CNN-based classifier

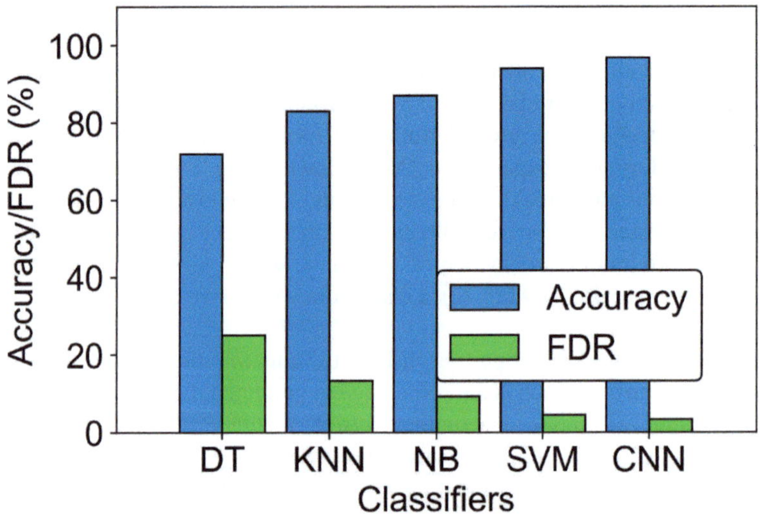

Fig. 5.6 Performance Comparison among four traditional machine learning and CNN-based classifier

overall recognition accuracy and FDR of five classifier. Our CNN-based method outperforms all four traditional methods and achieves 96.78% in recognition accuracy and 3.3% in FDR. We then show the dietary activity classification for five activities. As shown in Fig. 5.6, the recognition accuracy for all activities are higher than 90%. The accuracy of using bare hand is a little lower than other activities, because the body movement of using bare hand is similar to that of using spoon,

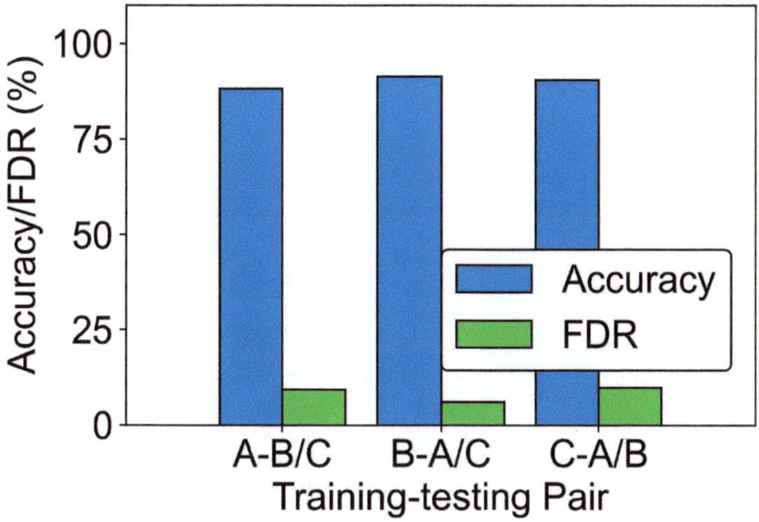

Fig. 5.7 Impact of environment on system performance

which may cause some confusion to the classifier. The result confirms that our CNN-based classifier can achieve robust performance in dietary activity classification.

5.5.3 Impact of Different Environments

We then evaluate the impact of different environments on system performance. In particular, we collect data from three different environments mentioned in Sect. 5.5.1. We use data from one environment as the training set and data from the other two environments as the testing set and try different training-testing pairs. As demonstrated in Fig. 5.7, all of the training-testing pairs achieve classification accuracy over 88% and with FDR below 9% even the training set and testing set are collected from different places. This result proves that our system is able to offer domain-invariant performance under different environments.

5.5.4 Impact of Monitoring Device Positions

Different positions of the device may affect the accuracy of dietary activity classification. We study the impact of device position on our CNN-based classifier. We evaluate three positions demonstrated in Fig. 5.4. As shown in Fig. 5.8, at all three positions, our system maintains an FDR lower than 4%. The accuracy of position P1 and position P2 are slightly lower than that of default position S.

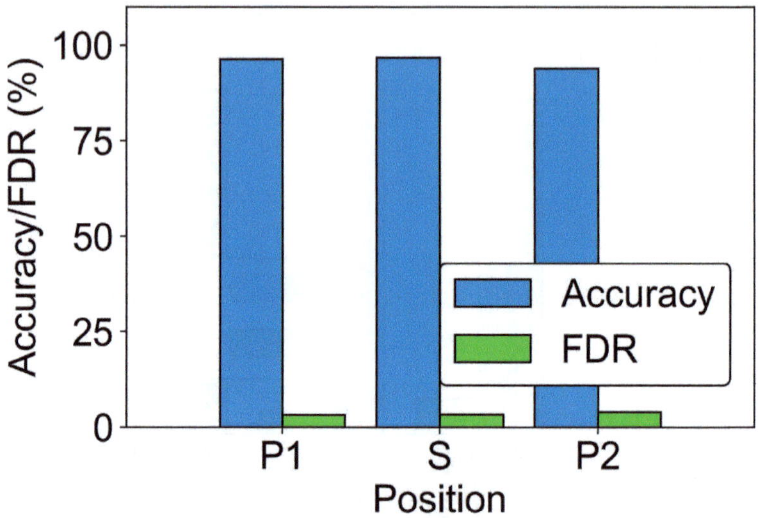

Fig. 5.8 Impact of different positions of mmWave device in office

This is because when the device is located at a position not facing the user, user's arms are parallel to the device, causing weaker Doppler effects and vaguer Spatial-Temporal Heatmaps. But our system still maintains an accuracy over 94%. The result proves that our system can still maintain a good performance in dietary activity classification even the device is situated at different positions. We also test the system at three distances (i.e., 1, 1.5, 2 m) at position S and find that the performance is not affected.

5.5.5 System Performance of Eating Period Estimation

We next evaluate the performance of eating period estimation for different food intake activities. In our experiments, each of the 5 activities is performed 160 times and we collected 800 eating activities in total. As shown in Fig. 5.9, the average estimated error (indicated by red points) of using fork, fork&knife, spoon, chopsticks and bare hand are 67, 88, 141, 67 and 124 ms, respectively, which are all within 150 ms. Additionally, the estimated error for all the collected activities are all smaller than 400 ms. The results demonstrate that our proposed system can precisely estimate eating period and maintain a low estimated error for different activities. Furthermore, by calculating the average time duration of each eating activity, we can estimate users' eating speed and infer high-level information such as calories intake or analysis of nutritional balance. The detailed dietary information can be further used to assist the healing of various health problems caused by bad eating habits.

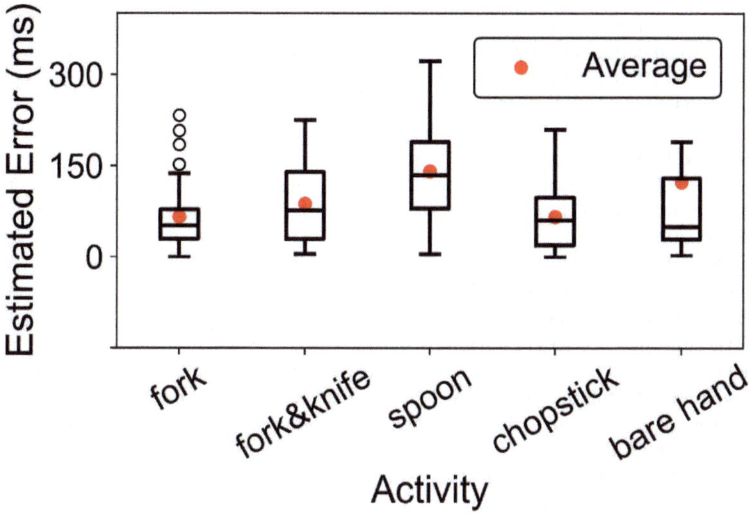

Fig. 5.9 Comparison of eating period estimated error

5.6 Summary

In this chapter, we demonstrate the feasibility of using mmWave signals for detailed dietary behavior monitoring. Our proposed system utilizes a CNN-based approach, exhibiting robustness to varied environments without necessitating additional training. By providing a comprehensive understanding of eating behaviors, the system equips users with insights to rectify unhealthy dietary habits. The extensive experimental results affirm the efficacy of our system, with an average accuracy exceeding 97.5% in dietary activity recognition and a false detection rate of less than 5%.

References

1. Amft, O.: A wearable earpad sensor for chewing monitoring. In: Sensors, 2010, pp. 222–227. IEEE (2010). https://doi.org/10.1109/ICSENS.2010.5690449
2. CDC: The harmful effects of poor nutrition (2024). https://www.cdc.gov/chronicdisease/resources/publications/factsheets/nutrition.htm
3. Cspinet: Why good nutrition is important (2017). https://www.cspinet.org/eating-healthy/why-good-nutrition-important
4. Kong, F., Tan, J.: Dietcam: automatic dietary assessment with mobile camera phones. Pervasive Mobile Comput. **8**, 147–163 (2012). https://doi.org/10.1016/j.pmcj.2011.07.003
5. Lin, Z., Xie, Y., Guo, X., Ren, Y., Chen, Y., Wang, C.: Wieat: fine-grained device-free eating monitoring leveraging wi-fi signals. In: 2020 29th International Conference on Computer Communications and Networks (ICCCN), pp. 1–9 (2020). https://doi.org/10.1109/ICCCN49398.2020.9209628

6. Ohkuma, T., Hirakawa, Y., Nakamura, U., Kiyohara, Y., Kitazono, T., Ninomiya, T.: Association between eating rate and obesity: a systematic review and meta-analysis. Int. J. Obesity **39**(11), 1589–1596 (2015)
7. O'Loughlin, G., Cullen, S.J., McGoldrick, A., O'Connor, S., Blain, R., O'Malley, S., Warrington, G.D.: Using a wearable camera to increase the accuracy of dietary analysis (2013). https://doi.org/10.1016/j.amepre.2012.11.007
8. Raja, M., Vali, Z., Palipana, S., Michelson, D.G., Sigg, S.: 3d head motion detection using millimeter-wave doppler radar. IEEE Access **8**, 32321–32331 (2020). https://doi.org/10.1109/ACCESS.2020.2973957
9. Ren, Y., Lu, J., Beletchi, A., Huang, Y., Karmanov, I., Fontijne, D., Patel, C., Xu, H.: Hand gesture recognition using 802.11ad mmwave sensor in the mobile device. In: 2021 IEEE Wireless Communications and Networking Conference Workshops (WCNCW), pp. 1–6 (2021). https://doi.org/10.1109/WCNCW49093.2021.9419978
10. Schubert, E., Sander, J., Ester, M., Kriegel, H.P., Xu, X.: Dbscan revisited, revisited: why and how you should (still) use dbscan. ACM Trans. Database Syst. (TODS) **42**(3), 1–21 (2017)
11. Simonyan, K., Zisserman, A.: Very deep convolutional networks for large-scale image recognition. In: International Conference on Learning Representations (2015)
12. Wang, Y., Liu, J., Chen, Y., Gruteser, M., Yang, J., Liu, H.: E-eyes: device-free location-oriented activity identification using fine-grained wifi signatures. In: Proceedings of the 20th Annual International Conference on Mobile Computing and Networking, MobiCom '14, p. 617–628. Association for Computing Machinery, New York (2014). https://doi.org/10.1145/2639108.2639143
13. Zhang, S., Ang, Jr., M.H., Xiao, W., Tham, C.K.: Detection of activities by wireless sensors for daily life surveillance: eating and drinking. Sensors **9**, 1499–517 (2009). https://doi.org/10.3390/s90301499

Chapter 6
Fitness Assistance Using Motion Sensor

Motion sensors are now a standard feature on most wearables and smartphones, providing a consistent and portable tracking solution across diverse settings even in varied environments. Acknowledging the transformative impact of these sensors in enhancing users' lifestyles (e.g., sleep monitoring and running rhythm tracking), this chapter explores a virtual fitness coach leveraging users' wearable mobile devices (including wrist-worn wearables and arm-mounted smartphones) to assess dynamic postures (movement patterns and positions) in workouts. Our system aims to help users achieve effective workout and prevent injury by dynamically depicting the short-term and long-term picture of their workout based on various sensors in wearable mobile devices. In particular, the system recognizes different types of exercises and interprets fine-grained fitness data (i.e., motion strength and speed) to an easy-to-understand exercise review score, which provides a comprehensive workout performance evaluation and recommendation. The system has the ability to align the sensor readings from wearable devices to the human coordinate system, ensuring the accuracy and robustness of the system. Extensive experiments with over 5000 repetitions of 12 types of exercises involve 12 participants doing both anaerobic and aerobic exercises in indoors as well as outdoors. Our results demonstrate that our system can provide meaningful review and recommendations to users by accurately measure their workout performance and achieve 93% accuracy for workout analysis.

The reminder of this chapter is organized as follows. In Sect. 6.1, we present the research background. In Sect. 6.2, we review existing work in the field. Section 6.4 discusses the system design for fitness assistance using motion sensors. Section 6.5 provides detailed information on system implementation. The system evaluation will be covered in Sect. 6.6. Finally, we conclude the chapter with a summary in Sect. 6.7.

X. Guo et al., *Mobile Technologies for Smart Healthcare System Design*, Wireless Networks, https://doi.org/10.1007/978-3-031-57345-3_6

6.1 Background

The proliferation of *wearable mobile devices* (e.g., smartwatches, wrist-worn fitness bands, and smartphones mounted on arms) has already shown its potential on improving our life styles through a great number of applications in smart healthcare, smart home, and smart cities. An important use case of wearable mobile devices is providing guidelines to improve people's daily activities, for example, tracking walking steps [13], monitoring sleep qualities [9], and estimating daily caloric intake [10]. In this work, we take one step further by answering the question: Whether such wearable mobile devices become powerful enough in leveraging fine-grained sensing information to perform systematic comprehensive fitness assistance and prevent injuries.

Traditionally, fitness monitoring is performed by analyzing the workout captured by video tapes [2] or specialized sensors [3, 4]. Chang et al. [3] track free-weight exercises by incorporating an accelerometer into a workout glove. Cheng et al. [4] develop a technique that can recognize human activities by attaching a sensor on users' hips. In recent years, smartphone apps, fitness trackers and dedicated devices, such as Sworkit (http://sworkit.com/), Fitbit (https://www.fitbit.com/), Garmin watch (http://www.garmin.com/en-US/) and Gym watch (https://www.gymwatch.com/), show the initial success of fitness monitoring. They can perform step counts and log exercises based on users' manual inputs. Additionally, people need to purchase dedicated sensors and wear them during exercises. Hao et al. [7] present a system using smartphone and its external microphone that detects running rhythm and improves exercise efficiency for runners. Yet the question whether or not mobile devices can automatically distinguish different types of exercises and provide fine-grained performance recommendation related to exercises remains open.

Toward this end, we search for an integrated mobile solution that can perform systematic fitness monitoring and performance review. We propose leveraging wearable mobile devices to achieve the following two main aspects:

(i) **Fine-grained Fitness Data Interpretation.** Recording the sensor readings on wearable mobile devices (e.g., smartwatch or smartphone) during workout to explore their capability of deriving fine-grained exercise information including exercise types, the number of set and the number of repetitions (reps) per set. The derived quantitative data can be further analyzed for inferring meaningful information. For example, higher level information can be obtained including calories burn, body fat, body mass index, etc.

(ii) **Smart Exercise Guidance.** Furthermore, the derived fitness data is of great importance to assist the users to maintain proper exercise postures and avoid injuries. To build muscles and gain a healthier body, it is widely recognized that people should perform their workout properly and effectively. Our system aims to not only regulate the workouts by following the Frequency, Intensity, Time and Type (FITT) principle [1], but also provide detailed guidelines to review the user's posture through workout and provide recommendation in keeping correct exercise form (e.g., in terms of speed of exercise execution and strength).

In particular, the system exploits *Short Time Energy* (STE) to derive fine-grained fitness data (i.e., strength and speed of body movements) in exercises and recognizes different types of exercises automatically by using embedded sensors (e.g., accelerometer and gyroscope) on wearable mobile devices. Rooted in the understanding of body movements in exercises, our system develops a novel metric for evaluating the quality of each user's exercises, *exercise-form score*. This score reflects the difference of strength and speed of body movements between each repetition of an exercise based on a reference profile. The reference profile could be either obtained from the user's own sensor data or built from other people's data (e.g., training coaches or members from the same fitness club) through crowdsourcing platforms (e.g., fitness club's facebook, WhatsApp or WeChat).

The contributions of our work are summarized as follows. Our system aims to provide comprehensive benefits for workout analysis and performance evaluation. It includes assessing dynamic postures automatically during both anaerobic and aerobic exercises, achieving precise exercise recognition without user involvement, calculating exercise form scores, and offering performance reviews to enhance the quality of workouts and prevent injuries in the short and long term. To ensure accurate recognition, the sensing data is aligned into the human coordinate system, accommodating different device and exercise orientations. The system's performance has been demonstrated using smartwatches and mobile phones in armbands, achieving an high accuracy of for workout analysis in various gym and outdoor settings.

6.2 Related Work

Recent studies show that life experience can be improved through implementing various types of techniques using sensors and wireless technologies including activity recognition [4, 11, 12, 15, 17, 18] and physical exercises monitoring [3, 6, 7, 11].

There has been active work for activity recognition, including daily activities [4, 11, 17] and healthcare related activities such as eating [15] and smoking [12]. Vlasic et al. [17] develop a full body motion capture system by using multiple sensors attached on a human body. Cheng et al. [4] develop a technique that can recognize activities without training by placing a sensor on users' hips. These studies show that either external sensors or sensors embedded in wearables have the capability to accurately recognize human daily activities. Furthermore, video-based technologies can capture and recognize human hand motion [14] but require line-of-sight.

Another aspect of related studies focus on automatically monitoring physical exercises. There are mobile Apps (http://sworkit.com/), wristband (https://www.fitbit.com/) and solutions based on mobile devices with sensors [3, 6, 7, 11]. Chang et al. [3] propose to track free weight exercises by incorporating an accelerometer into a workout glove. In addition, Ding et al. [6] propose to recognize free-weight activities by attaching passive RFID tags on the dumbbells. Along this line, Hao et al. [7] propose to monitor the running rhythm by measuring breathing and strides with headsets and smartphones. These techniques rely on additional sensors or specific hardware. Most importantly, whether a workout feedback and guidance can be further provided to improve exercise performance still an open question.

The commercial products also exhibit the trend to automate the fitness monitoring, such as Garmin watch (http://www.garmin.com/en-US/) and Gym watch (https://www.gymwatch.com/). However, Garmin watch requires explicit inputs from users, including the type of workout and the start/stop time. Gym watch requires people to purchase dedicated sensors and wear them during exercises. Along this trend, the proposed system utilizes existing wearable devices (e.g., wrist-worn smartwatches or arm-mounted smartphones) to automatically provide fine-grained tracking of workout and offer exercise review and guidance to improve fitness experience.

6.3 Fitness Assistance via Embedded Motion Sensors in Wearable Devices

6.3.1 Design Challenges and Practical Issues

Exercise Form Correction Using Single Wearable Mobile Device It is necessary for the system to understand the performance of a exercise through the body movements, which is a challenging task to cope with by using a single wearable mobile device. This is because commercial mobile devices usually have limited low-power sensing modalities (i.e., accelerometer, gyroscope and magnetometer). Therefore, the system needs to be designed in such a way that can provide exercise form corrections based on the dynamics of sensor data resulted from the partial knowledge of the exercises.

Robust Fine-grained Exercise Differentiation It is also challenging to utilize sensors in wearable mobile devices to correctly distinguish different types of exercises, since sensor readings collected from the wearable mobile devices are extremely noisy due to the dynamic nature of exercises. Thus, it is important to devise a robust exercise classifier that can eliminate the impact of noisy sensor data and capture the fine-grained differences between different types of exercises.

Automated Wearing Orientation Alignment During exercises, wearable mobile devices may change its facing from the original direction from time to time. Such orientation changes result in unstable projection of user's body movements in the mobile device's coordinate system. This makes it hard for the system to determine the pattern of body movements. Therefore, a light-weight alignment algorithm is needed to transform the sensor data to that in a stable orientation to facilitate accurate exercise recognition.

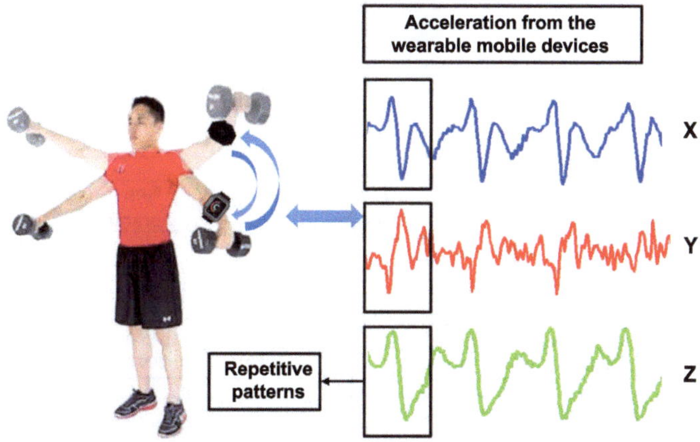

Fig. 6.1 Movement in exercises can be revealed by repetitive patterns from sensor readings of wearable mobile devices

6.3.2 Motion Sensor-based Fitness Monitoring System Design

The main goal of our system is to examine the users' dynamics (i.e., body movement patterns & intensities) in workouts and provide detailed workout statistics to assist users to achieve effective workouts and prevent injuries.

Given that these wearable mobile devices are worn on the human body of either wrist or upper arm, they become desirable interfaces to sense exercise movements to provide detailed workout statistics/analysis.

As illustrated in Fig. 6.1, the repetitive pattern of body movements in exercises can be well captured by using the inertial sensors of the wearable mobile device (i.e., a smartwatch). The system can automatically extract fine-grained fitness information (e.g., basic statistics, motion energy and performing period) without users' cooperation and provides users with illustrative feedback, which can also be exploited to enforce the Frequency, Intensity, Time, Type (FITT) principle of training [1].

As illustrated in Fig. 6.2, our system takes time-series of sensor readings as input from accelerometer and gyroscope as well as quaternion, all of which are readily available in off-the-shelf wearable mobile devices. We first perform *Workout Detection* to filter out the sensor readings that don't contain workout activities based on the presence of periodicity pattern in workout activity. The sensor readings that are found to contain workout activities will be served to two tasks, *Workout Interpretation & Recognition* and *Workout Review/Recommendation*. The Workout Recognition performs quantitative analysis to the sensor readings and identify different types of workouts based on the acceleration features that can capture unique repetitive patterns of different exercises. The Workout Review/Recommendation examines the characteristics of each rep (i.e., energy and time intervals) and provides the novel exercise form scores as feedback to users for performance evaluation.

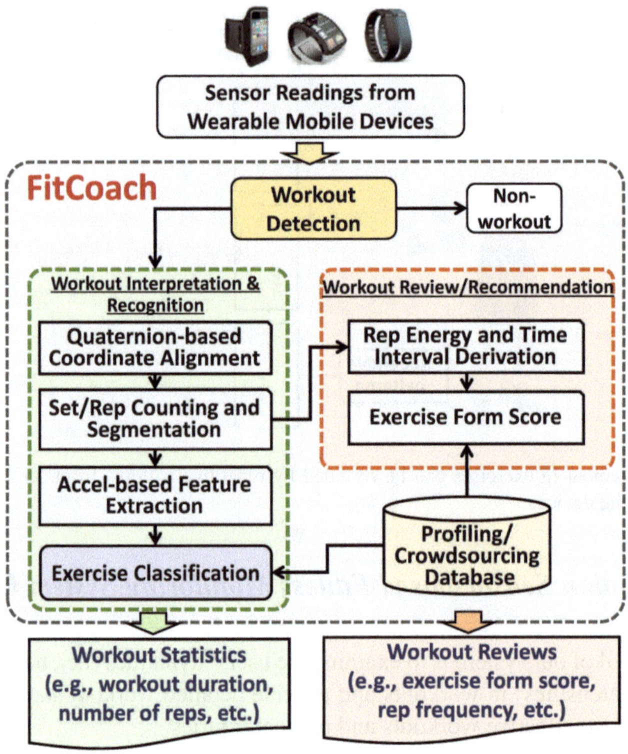

Fig. 6.2 The framework of the proposed fitness assistant system using motion sensor

Particularly, the Workout Recognition consists of four major components: *Quaternion-based Coordinate Alignment*, *Set/Rep Counting and Segmentation*, *Accel-based Feature Extraction*, and *Exercise Classification*. The Quaternion-based Coordinate Alignment tackles the issue of dynamic orientation in workouts, and automatically rotates sensor readings to a fixed coordinate system. The Set/Rep Counting counts the number of sets during the workout and the number of reps in each set based on the magnitude of the repetitive signals resulted from workouts. The sensor readings are further divided into small segments corresponding to the detected reps. In each segment, the Accel-based Feature Extraction derives statistics features that capture each repetitive moving patterns of exercises from three-axis acceleration readings. After Workout Interpretation, the system performs *Exercise Classification*, which utilizes a profile based algorithm to determine the types of exercises by comparing the extracted features with those of pre-collected profiles in the *Profiling/Crowdsourcing Database*.

In addition, the Workout Review/Recommendation aims to provide users with systematic fitness monitoring and performance review, which would assist the users to maintain proper exercise gestures and avoid injuries. The proposed system takes the segments of sensor readings identified in the Set/Rep Counting and

Segmentation as inputs, and performs the *Rep Energy and Time Interval Derivation* to estimate the characteristics of body movements in exercises (i.e., strength and frequency of the repetitive motions). The estimated characteristics are further utilized by the *Exercise Form Score Calculation* to calculate the exercise form score for each rep, which is a novel metric that allows the users to easily understand their performance in the exercises.

6.3.3 Fine-grained Workout Interpretation and Recognition

6.3.3.1 Workout Detection Using Autocorrelation

A key observation is that most regular exercises involve repetitive arm movements. For example, jogging and walking involve periodic arm swing, and weight lifting involves periodic pushing-ups. Such repetitive arm movements result in regularly changing values in sensor readings. In addition, the repetitive patterns from exercises tend to be last for a long time period simply because people normally adopt a set-and-rep scheme in exercise to maximize the effectiveness. Compared to regular exercises, non-workout activities usually don't have such long-term repetitive pattern. Therefore, we propose to detect workout based on determining whether there are long-term repetitive patterns in the sensor readings.

Towards this end, we adopt an autocorrelation-based approach to examine the accelerations resulted from exercise motions. The autocorrelation approach is a common technique used for detecting repetitive patterns in a time series. In particular, we first apply a moving time window with the length of w to the time series of accelerometer readings. For each time window, we use the Magnitude of Linear Acceleration (MLA) to estimate the linear acceleration (i.e., acceleration without gravitational acceleration) of exercise motions. The MLA based on accelerometer readings can be derived by the following equation:

$$MLA(i) = \sqrt{(a(i)_x)^2 + (a(i)_y)^2 + (a(i)_z)^2} - g, \tag{6.1}$$

where $a(i)_x$, $a(i)_y$ and $a(i)_z$ are the acceleration of the ith sample on the x, y and z axis of the mobile device respectively and g is the acceleration of gravity. Note that, the MLA in Eq. (6.1) equals to zero when there is no motion.

Then we calculate the autocorrelation of the time series of MLA, and use a typical peak finding algorithm [9] to find the number of peaks in the autocorrelation, which is denoted as N_p. The number of detected repetitive patterns thus can be derived with $N_r = (N_p - 1)/2$, due to the symmetric nature of the autocorrelation. Finally, to accommodate the noisy accelerometer readings, we use a threshold-based method to confirm the detected repetitive patterns are resulted from workouts. The workout detection results for each window can be derived by:

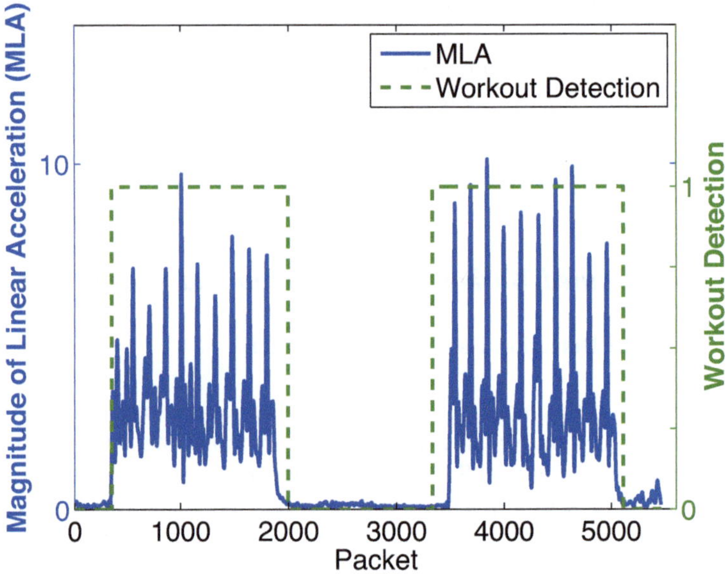

Fig. 6.3 Workout detection based on a 5-second sliding window (output 1 if the number of repetitive patterns is larger than 3 within the window, otherwise output 0)

$$D_w = \begin{cases} 1, & N_r > \nu \\ 0, & otherwise, \end{cases} \tag{6.2}$$

where D_w is a boolean value depicts whether the given sensor readings within a window belong to workout or not. D_w outputs 1 when N_r is bigger than a threshold value ν. Figure 6.3 shows an example of our workout detection results with $w = 5$s and $\nu = 3$, which demonstrates that our system can accurately detect the windows containing workouts.

6.3.3.2 Set/Repetition Segmentation Based on STE Analysis

After the Workout Detection, the system integrates the windows that are continuously labeled as workouts into a segment. The time between any two segments are identified as the rest interval, which will be provided as a part of the exercise review. However, in order to provide fine-grained exercise performance information, our system needs to look into the data in each set and analyzes the data based on a finer-grained concept, *repetition/rep*.

We devise a motion-energy-oriented approach to accurately estimate starting and ending time point of each repetition of the same exercise motion within a set. The intuition behind the approach is that each repetition usually consists of a series of arm movements that result in a unique pattern in terms of the accumulated motion

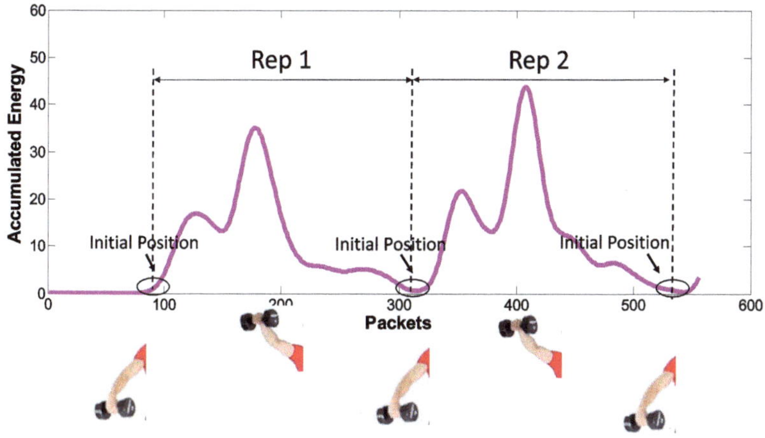

Fig. 6.4 Illustration of the relationship between the arm movements in a repetition and the unique pattern of accumulated energy captured by a wearable mobile device (i.e., a smartphone in an armband)

energy: (1) the accumulated energy starts to increase sharply from zero when the arm moves from an initial position to an ending position; (2) the accumulated energy drops a little when the arm pauses at the ending position for a very short while; (3) the accumulated energy starts to increase sharply again when the arm moves back from the ending position to the initial position; and (4) finally the accumulated energy drops sharply when the hand stops at the initial position for some rest. We found that this unique pattern of accumulated motion energy can be captured by the wearable mobile device through the Short Time Energy of MLA. Figure 6.4 illustrates the relationship of the unique pattern in the accumulated energy and the arm movements in each repetition.

Particularly, we adopt the Short Time Energy (STE) [5] to capture the unique energy pattern in the time series of MLA. The basic idea of this step is to accumulate the energy of the MLA in short sliding windows.

After obtaining STE of MLA, the system applies the same peak finding algorithm to detect the peaks in STE. Then the system finds the local minimum point between two peaks as the ending point of each repetition, and the data between two detected ending points are defined as a segment of repetition. Figure 6.5 shows an example of determining the repetition segments based on the local minimum points that are detected in STE of MLA from a wearable mobile device (i.e., a smartwatch) when the user conducts 3 sets of dumbbell rasing with 10 repetitions per set. The results indicate that the motion-energy-based approach can accurately separate the data for each repetition.

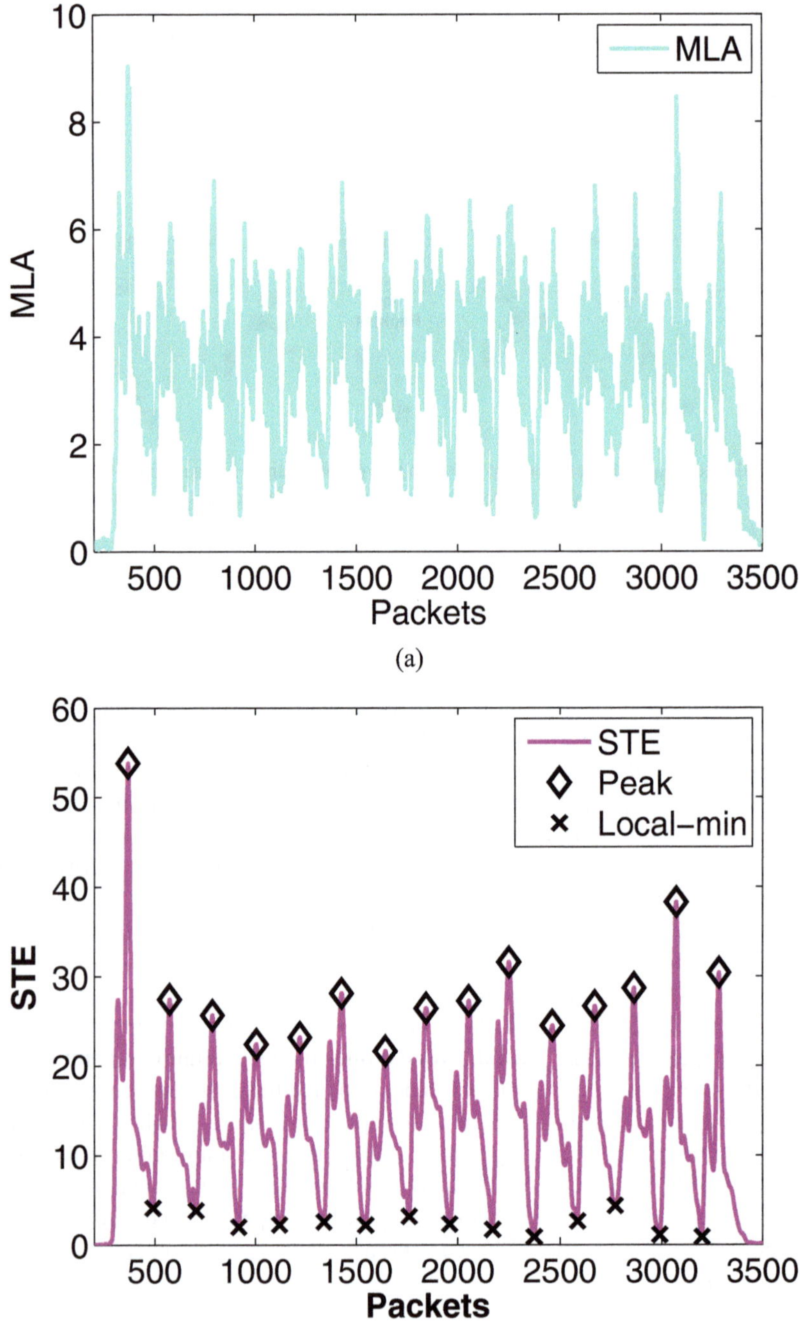

(a)

(b)

Fig. 6.5 Example of rep segmentation for 10 repetitions of dumbbell raising exercise. (**a**) Magnitude of Linear Acceleration (MLA). (**b**) Local minimum identified in Short Time Energy (STE) of MLA

6.3.3.3 Feature Extraction and Workout Classification

After repetition segmentation, the system aims to identify the workout type for each set. The basic idea is to build a database with the profiles for different types of workouts before the workout classification, then we use a profile-based approach to determine the workout type for each rep segment in the set, and further to infer the workout type of the entire set.

Accel-based Feature Extraction In order to distinguish different types of workouts, we need to find the features that can capture the unique characteristics of each type of workouts. Based on our extensive feature selection studies, we finally determine nine statistical acceleration-based features that are most useful to distinguish different types of workouts, namely *skewness, kurtosis, standard deviation, variance, most frequently appear in the array, median, range, trimmean and mean*. To extract features without worrying about the variation of the mobile device's facing orientation, we first perform the earth-reference alignment to rotate all acceleration data to the earth coordinate system. After the world-reference alignment, our system extracts the nine acceleration-based features from the already aligned three-axis accelerations in each rep segment to describe the body movements. In total, we extract 27 features (i.e., nine features per axis) for each rep segment.

Light-weight Classifier The proposed system utilizes a light-weight machine learning based approach to identify different types of workouts based on the acceleration-based features extracted from each rep segment. It is light-weight because the system only needs to determine the workout type for the first few rep segments within a set, and the workout type of the entire set of repetitions is identified as the majority decision based on the classification results from the first few rep segments. Specifically, we adopt a Support Vector Machine (SVM) classifier [16] with radial basis function kernel. The classifier is trained by the pre-collected profiles of different types of workouts.. We note that we utilize the classification results of the first five reps to determine the workout type of the entire set.

6.4 Workout Review and Recommendation

In order to achieve effective workouts and avoid injuries, users usually seek out personal fitness plans provided by fitness trainers or professionals. Such fitness plans often try to regulate the workouts by following the Frequency, Intensity, Time and Type (FITT) principle of training, which is a set of guidelines that instruct users to set up workout routines fitting their goals and fitness levels while maximizing the effects of exercises. However, most of users cannot afford a full-time personal trainer that can coach their workouts at any time. The system fills the gap between users and the fitness plans based on FITT principle of training by providing fine-grained fitness information and intuitive feedback to users. Specifically, the proposed system is able to track the following basic workout statistics automatically including *exercise type, number of reps, number of sets, time between sets, time between sessions (training days/week)* to enforce the FITT principle of training. In addition, our system further provides fine-grained feedback, which is the *exercise form score* in terms of motion energy and performance period for individual rep, to assist users in fine-tuning their exercises gestures.

6.4.1 Exercise Form Score Design

Besides providing basic workout statistics to the users, the system aims to offer users a more intuitive way to understand their performance in exercises by comparing their exercise statistics to a baseline, which could be either generated based on the users' own data or based on the data from croudsourcing. Towards this end, we define a novel metric named *exercise form score*, which consists of two subscores that respectively evaluate a user's fine-grained performance of each rep in the exercise based on two important criteria as shown below:

Motion Strength (MS) A proper exercise form should maintain the motion strength at a certain level. For example, too much strength may indicate that the user spend more energy on each rep and if the weight is too heavy, it will increase the risk of injury while too little strength may indicate that the user spend too less energy to build muscle effectively. We intuitively utilize the energy level of each rep to describe the motion strength, which mean a set of reps with good performance should maintain a stable energy level. The energy level of each rep can be estimated by the maximum value in obtained STE of MLA.

Performing Period (PP) A proper exercise form should avoid too-fast or too-slow movements in order to effectively build muscles and prevent injuries. In this work, we utilize the time period of each rep to describe the performing period of each rep, which reflects how fast a user performs a repetition in exercises. Therefore, a set of reps with good performance should also have similar time periods. The time period of each rep can be directly obtained from the length of each rep segment after the segmentation. We note that the performing period provides more insights to users. For example, users can leverage such information for equipment weight adjustment (e.g., reduced speed of last few reps in a set indicates that the user may be training exhausted and need to decrease the weight or number of reps in next set).

Exercise Form Score Based on these two criteria, the system defines the *Exercise Form Score*, which consists of two subscores: *MS score* and *PP score*. The subscores depict how the testing rep deviates from the baseline in terms of the motion strength and performing period, respectively. We discuss the details about the baseline in the next subsection. Particularly, the MS score for the ith rep is defined as:

$$E_i = \frac{A(i) - A^*}{A^*}, \quad i = 1, 2, 3, \ldots, n, \tag{6.3}$$

where $A(i)$ is the maximum STE of the MLA of the ith rep, and A^* is the motion strength baseline. Similarly, the PP score for the ith rep is defined as:

$$T_i = \frac{I(i) - I^*}{I^*}, \quad i = 1, 2, 3, \ldots, n, \tag{6.4}$$

where I_i is the length of the ith rep and I^* is the performing period baseline. The output exercise form score is a 2-tuple score that can be denoted as $< E_i, T_i >$.

The exercise form score reflects the performance of the testing rep comparing to a baseline. We design two baselines that are suitable in different scenarios, namely *Personal Baseline* and *Crowdsouring Baseline.*

Personal Baseline We observe that users usually can perform exercises with standard strength and frequency at the beginning of the workout, but the quality of the exercises decays with time due to fatigue. Based on this observation, a good candidate of the baseline for evaluating the performance of a user's workouts is the early portion of the user's own reps. In particular, we derive the personal baseline by averaging the motion strength and performing period of the first k reps of the first set in the user's sensor data. We empirically choose $k = 5$ in our work.

Crowdsourcing Baseline The personal baseline is good for short-term exercise performance evaluation but could be bias to the user's own preference. For example, a user could feel tired at the beginning of the exercise and result in bad baseline for evaluating the entire exercise. To tackle this problem, we further propose the crowdsourcing baseline, which allows users to compare their performance with the baseline from exemplars (e.g., fitness coaches, bodybuilders, and amateur expertise) to achieve a long-term and more accurate exercise performance evaluation. The crowdsourcing approach is feasible because it is an increasing trend that people would like to share their fitness data in online social network to earn credits or build record, and more social platforms, such as WhatsApp and WeChat, start to provide the functionality allowing people to share their fitness data among friends.

6.4.2 Workout Review Plane Design

The system further adopts an unique view angle of the exercise form score to allow users to track the performance or their each rep in a illustrative way. In particular, we define a *review plane* in which the x axis and y axis are the MS score and PP score, respectively. According to Eqs. (6.3) and (6.4), the Original represents the rep having the exactly same performance as the chosen baseline, and every exercise form score $< E_i, T_i >$ corresponding to the ith rep can be mapped to a position in the the review plane. Apparently, the rep having its position closer to the Original has better performance, and the more reps close to the Original the better.

Figures 6.6 and 6.7compares the workout reviews of two different users (i.e., User A an User B) in a set of lateral raising exercises (i.e., 15 reps in one set). Figures 6.6a and 6.7a respectively depict STE of MLA of two users' reps, which shows that User A has more stable energy levels and time lengths for each repetition than User B. Figures 6.6b and 6.7b respectively illustrate two users' exercise form scores based on their personal baselines in the review planes, which shows that the score points of User A are concentrated around the Original while the score points of User B are scattered around the second quadrant of the review plane. The observation indicates that User B have much higher motion strength and longer performing period comparing to the user's first few reps, and thus have worse performance than User A.

6.5 System Implementation

6.5.1 *Quaternion-based Coordinate Alignment*

In workout monitoring scenarios, users wearing wearable mobile devices basically involve three different coordinate systems as illustrated in Fig. 6.8, namely, *mobile device coordinate*, *earth coordinate*, and *human coordinate*. The sensor readings from a mobile device are defined in the device coordinate and thus result in non-fixed projection of the user's body movements defined in the human coordinate. In order to address this issue, the system adopts a quaternion-based approache to dynamically convert sensor readings from the mobile device coordinate either to the human coordinate or to a coordinate system having the fixed mapping to the human coordinate.

6.5.1.1 Earth-reference Alignment

For exercise recognition in a gym, the orientation of wearable mobile devices may change due to rotation caused by arm movement. Therefore, our system needs to convert sensor readings from the mobile device coordinate to the earth coordinate first. Specifically, we convert the sensor readings from the mobile device coordinate to the earth coordinate by using the quaternion-based rotation $p_e = q_{me} p_m q_{me}^{-1}$, where p_m is the sensor reading vector (e.g., accelerations) in the mobile device coordinate, and q_{me} is the quaternion reading from the mobile device coordinate to the earth coordinate, which can be obtained from the device directly. q_{me}^{-1} is the conjugate quaternion of q_{me}. After conversion, the converted sensor readings p_e are in the earth coordinate and can provide stable patterns of body movements during exercises to enable our exercise recognition.

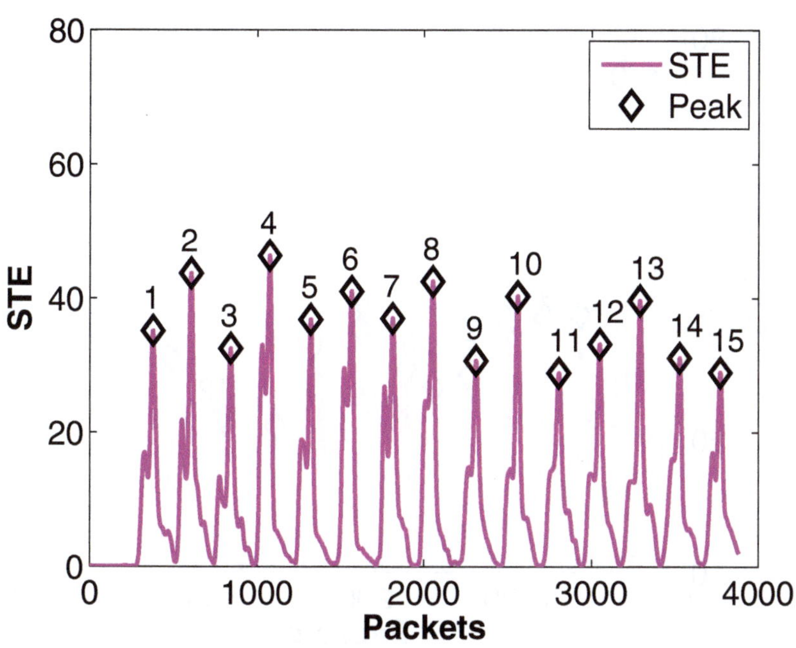

(a)

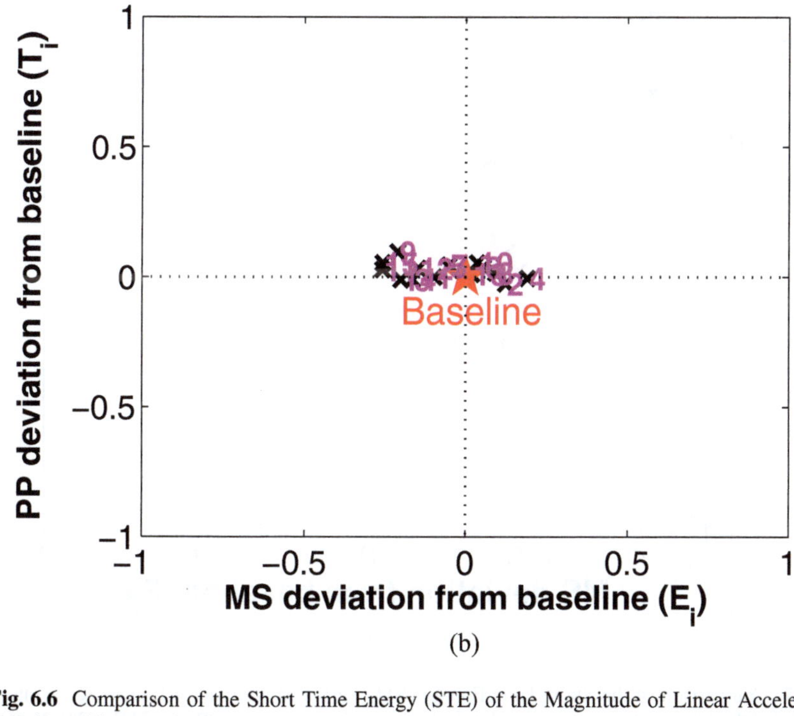

(b)

Fig. 6.6 Comparison of the Short Time Energy (STE) of the Magnitude of Linear Acceleration (MLA) and the exercise form scores on the workout review plane of user A. (**a**) STE of MLA, user A. (**b**) Exercise form scores on the workout review plan, user A

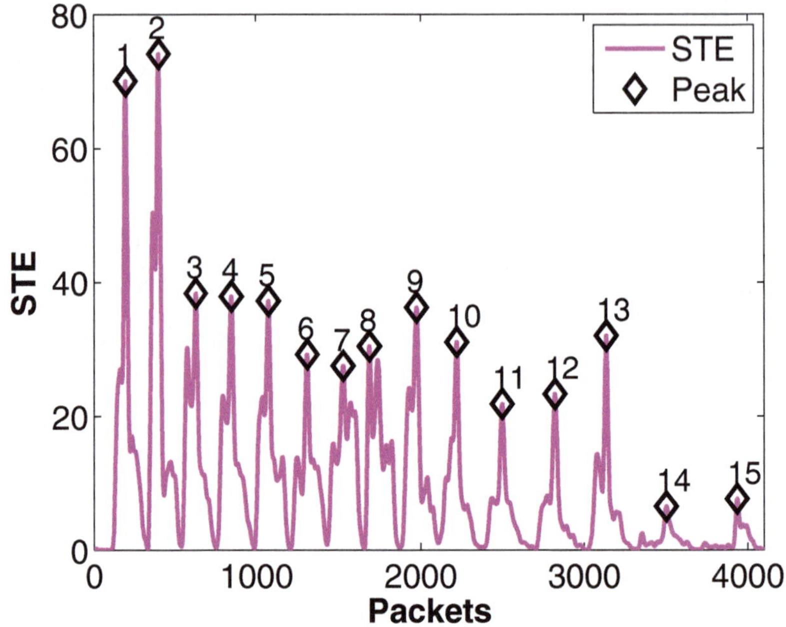

(a)

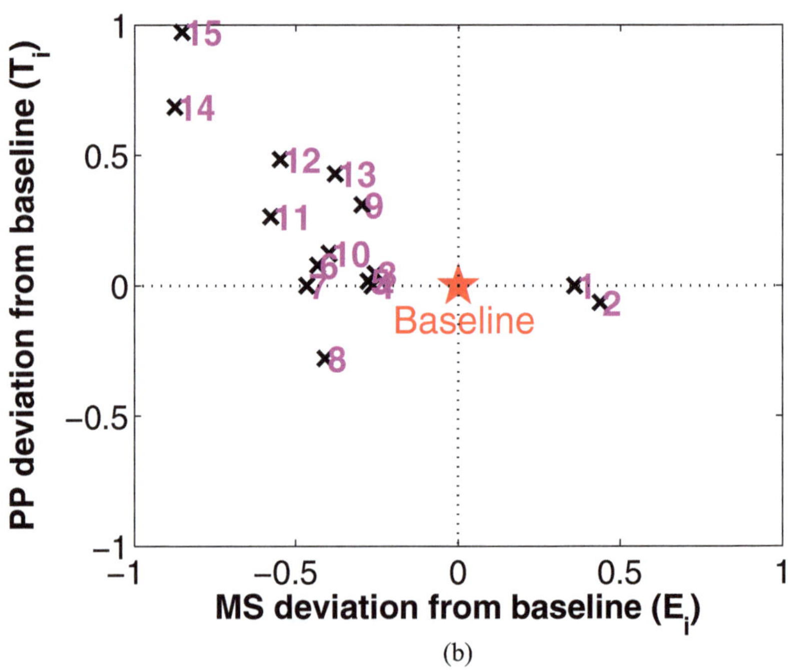

(b)

Fig. 6.7 Comparison of the Short Time Energy (STE) of the Magnitude of Linear Acceleration (MLA) and the exercise form scores on the workout review plane of user B. (**a**) STE of MLA, user B. (**b**) Exercise form scores on the workout review plan, user B

6.5.1.2 User-reference Alignment

We notice that using quaternion to align sensor reading from wearable coordinate to earth coordinate solves the different wearing orientation of wearable devices. Furthermore, we should also consider when people doing workout in gym with different facing directions.

Specifically, we convert the sensor readings from the mobile device coordinate to the human coordinate by using the quaternion-based rotation $p_h = q_{mh} p_m q_{mh}^{-1}$, where p_m and p_h is the sensor reading vector in the mobile device coordinate and the human coordinate respectively. q_{mh}^{-1} is the conjugate quaternion of q_{mh}, q_{mh} is the quaternion readings from the mobile device to the human coordinate, which can be calculated using Hamilton product: $q_{mh} = q_{he}^{-1} q_{me}$, where q_{me} is the quaternion reading from the mobile device coordinate to the earth coordinate, which can be obtained from the device directly. q_{he}^{-1} is the conjugate quaternion of q_{he}, and q_{he} is the quaternion readings from the human to the earth coordinate, which can be derived from the estimated facing direction.

More specifically, we can derive $q_{he} = [w, x, y, z]$ using the *Euler angles* in earth coordinate which is defined as:

$$
\begin{cases}
w = cos\left(\frac{\phi}{2}\right) cos\left(\frac{\theta}{2}\right) cos\left(\frac{\psi}{2}\right) - sin\left(\frac{\phi}{2}\right) sin\left(\frac{\theta}{2}\right) sin\left(\frac{\psi}{2}\right) \\
x = cos\left(\frac{\phi}{2}\right) sin\left(\frac{\theta}{2}\right) cos\left(\frac{\psi}{2}\right) + sin\left(\frac{\phi}{2}\right) cos\left(\frac{\theta}{2}\right) cos\left(\frac{\psi}{2}\right) \\
y = cos\left(\frac{\phi}{2}\right) sin\left(\frac{\theta}{2}\right) cos\left(\frac{\psi}{2}\right) - sin\left(\frac{\phi}{2}\right) cos\left(\frac{\theta}{2}\right) sin\left(\frac{\psi}{2}\right) \\
z = cos\left(\frac{\phi}{2}\right) cos\left(\frac{\theta}{2}\right) sin\left(\frac{\psi}{2}\right) + sin\left(\frac{\phi}{2}\right) sin\left(\frac{\theta}{2}\right) cos\left(\frac{\psi}{2}\right),
\end{cases}
\tag{6.5}
$$

where rotation angles ϕ, θ and ψ are the *row*, *pitch* and *yaw* respect to earth reference respectively as shown in Fig. 6.8. We assume that people are running on the horizontal ground and therefore ϕ and θ are equal to zero and we only need to calculate facing direction ψ (i.e., *yaw*).

6.5.2 Facing Direction Estimation

We observe that in rest time and aerobic exercises, the direction of the user's arm swing is usually in line with the user's facing direction, suggesting that we can exploit the arm swing direction to estimate the user's facing direction. For anaerobic exercise, users can simply swing their arms for a few times to assist the system for facing direction estimation.

In particular, the system segments each arm swing using rep segmentation, then converts the acceleration readings from mobile device's coordinate into earth

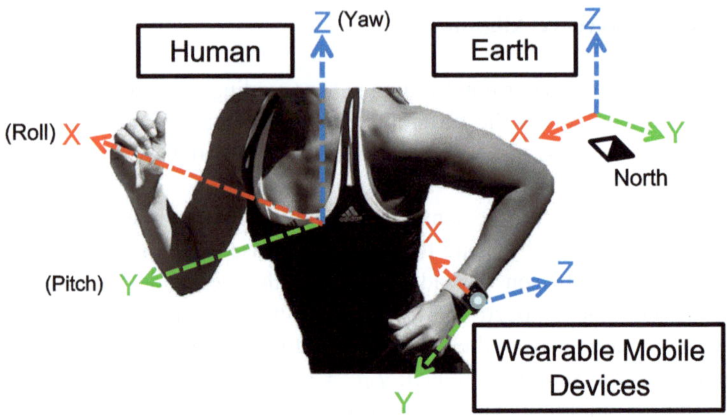

Fig. 6.8 Three coordinate systems

coordinate. After conversion, we can double integrate the acceleration projected to the x and y axes in the earth coordinate to derive the moving distance of the arm along the x and y axes, respectively. In this work, we define the arm swing direction as the counter-clockwise rotation around the z-axis from y-axis in the earth coordinate (i.e., North direction), which is similar to the definition of yaw in *Euler angles*. We first calculate the included angle δ between the displacement of x-axis and y-axis caused by arm swing by using $\delta = \left|arctan\left(s_y/s_x\right)\right|$, where s_x, s_y are the distance accumulated from acceleration in x-axis and y-axis respectively by using *Trapezoidal rule* [8]. Note that δ is ranging from 0° to 90° and then we need to convert it from 0° to 360°. Therefore, we need to decide the quadrant Q of arm swing direction, that is defined in Cartesian system where x and y are East and North in earth reference respectively, to convert it to ψ ranging from 0° to 360° as:

$$\psi = \begin{cases} 270^\circ + \delta; & if\ Q = 1, \\ 90^\circ - \delta; & if\ Q = 2, \\ 90^\circ + \delta; & if\ Q = 3, \\ 270^\circ - \delta; & if\ Q = 4, \end{cases} \tag{6.6}$$

where Q can be determined based on the order of maximum and minimum values (i.e., peak and trough) on x and y axes of accelerometer.

We evaluate the proposed facing direction estimation by asking a volunteer to run toward four different directions (i.e., north, south, east and west in earth reference). Figure 6.9 shows the 10-round estimation results for each direction. We find that the estimated results are along with the four running directions and good enough in the system, the little bias is caused by the fact that people swing their arms naturally while running which is not perfectly stick to their facing directions.

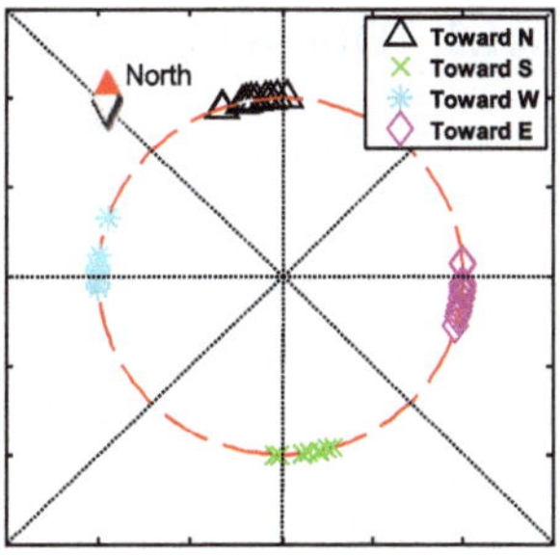

Fig. 6.9 Facing direction estimation of four running directions: toward North (N), South (S), West (W) and East (E)

6.5.3 Workout Profile Construction

When users start the system for the first time, they are asked to build a profile database for the exercise recognition by performing the particular types of exercises. The system extracts the accl-based features, and asks the user to manually label the corresponding exercise types. We note that proposed system allows users to wear the wearable mobile devices with flexible facing orientation when constructing the profiling database, because the quaternion-based coordinate alignment always converts sensor readings to a coordinate system that has the fixed mapping relationship to the human coordinate during exercises.

6.6 System Evaluation

In this section, we first present the experimental methodology and metrics we used to evaluate the proposed system. We then evaluate the performance and robustness of the system using both smartwatch and smartphone during people's fitness workout.

6.6.1 Experimental Methodology

6.6.1.1 Wearable Mobile Devices

We evaluate the system with two types of wearable mobile devices (i.e., a smartphone of Samsung Galaxy Note 3 and a smartwatch of LG Watch Urbane). Both devices use Android and can collect sensor readings of accelerometer, gyroscope and quaternion vector. In our experiment, the participants are asked to wear the smartwatch on the wrist with their own wearing preferences and the phone is mounted on their upper arms using a jogging armband. During exercise, sensor readings are collected with the sampling rate of 100 Hz. The ground truth of workout statistics are recorded by a volunteer.

6.6.1.2 Fitness Data Collection

We recruit 12 volunteers from colleagues, friends and students. Among them, 7 out of 12 go to gym regularly and the rest go to gym less frequently. For over a half year experiments, all 12 volunteers are asked to wear the smartwatch and smartphone simultaneously at the same arm, which is for the performance comparison between smartwatch and smartphone of the same exercise. In addition, a volunteer accompany with them to record the ground truth. Specifically, we study 12 different exercise types. The tested exercises include both anaerobic exercises, including weight machines and free weights, and aerobic exercises in which around 2 hours running is tested in both indoors (e.g., treadmill) and outdoors. In total, we collect over 5000 repetitions of 12 types of exercises involving 12 participants.

6.6.2 Evaluation Metrics

We use the following metrics to evaluate the proposed system:

Precision Given N_e reps of a exercise/ gesture type e in our collected data, precision of recognizing the exercise type e is defined as $Precision_e = N_e^T/(N_e^T + M_e^F)$,where N_e^T is the number of instances collectedly recognized as exercise e. M_e^F is the number of sets corresponding to other exercises that are mistakenly recognized as exercise e.

Recall Recall of the exercise type e is defined as the ratio of the reps that are correctly recognized as the exercise e over all reps of exercise type e. which is defined as $Recall_e = N_e^T/N_e$.

F1-Score F1-score is the harmonic mean of precision and recall, which reaches its best value at 1 and worst at 0. In our multi-class scenario, the F1-score for a specific gesture e was defined as $F_1^{(e)} = 2 \times \frac{precision_e \times recall_e}{precision_e + recall_e}$.

Repetition Detection Rate Given all reps of an exercise type e, rep detection rate is defined as the ratio of the number of detected reps of e over all reps of e the user performed.

6.6.3 Workout Recognition Using Smartwatch

We first evaluate the performance of our system on exercise recognition using smartwatch. Figure 6.10a shows the confusion matrix of the recognizing exercise types by using smartwatch. An entry M_{ij} denotes the percentage between the number of exercise i was predicted as gesture j and the total number of i. The average accuracy is 95% with standard deviation 5% over all 12 types of exercises.

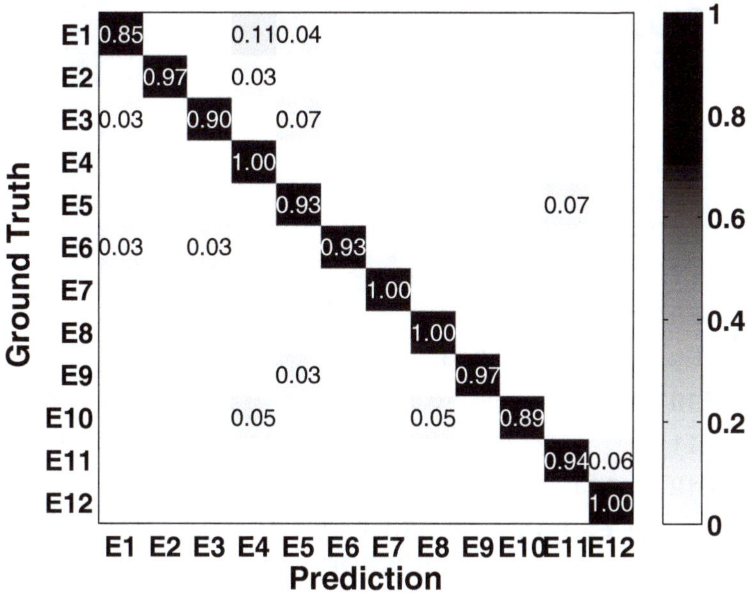

(a)

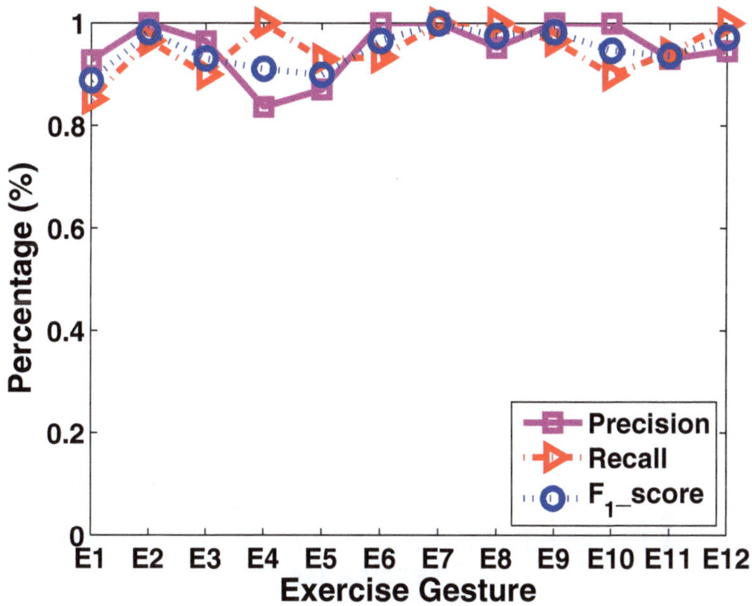

(b)

Fig. 6.10 Comparison of the performance of recognizing 12 exercises between using a smartwatch and a smartphone. (**a**) Confusion matrix, smartwatch. (**b**) Precision/recall/F1 score, smartwatch. (**c**) Confusion matrix, smartphone. (**d**) Precision/recall/F1 score, smartphone

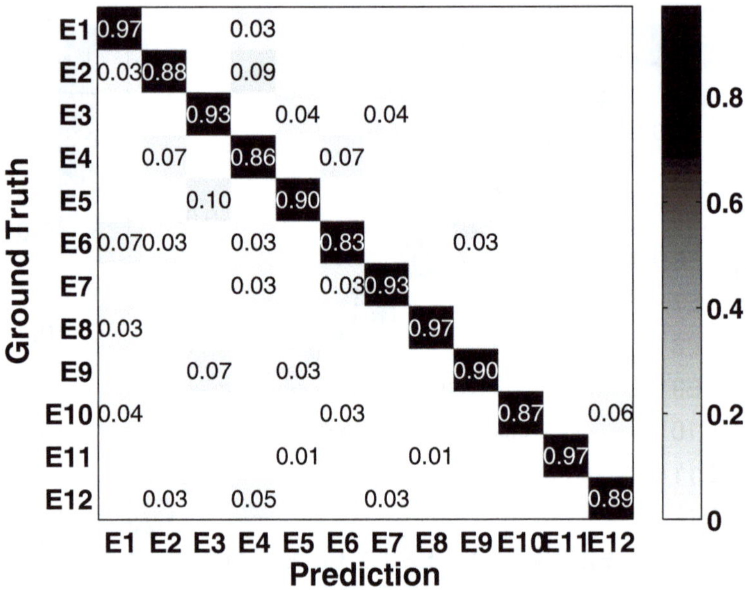

(c)

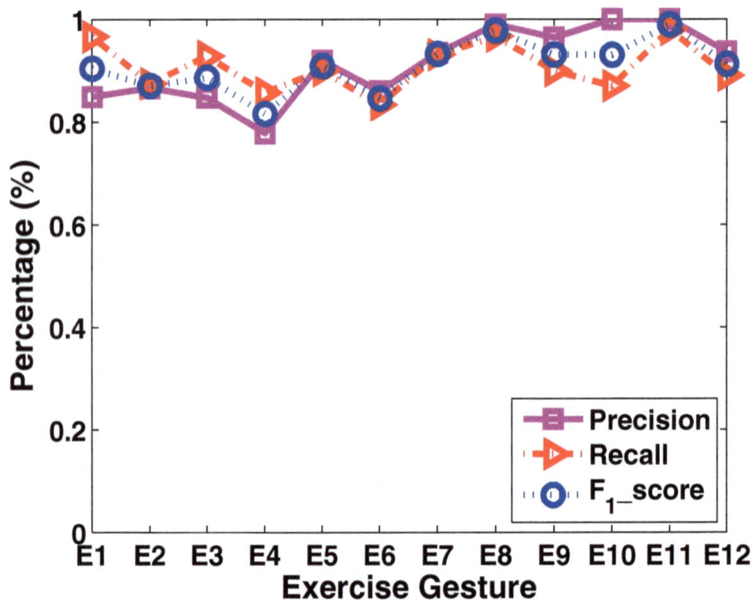

(d)

Fig. 6.10 (continued)

We find that recognizing results from $E1$ and $E10$ are relatively low, which are 85 and 89% respectively. This may be caused by some volunteers who go to gym less frequently and cannot maintain the exercise in a correct form for all reps. For example, $E10$ (i.e., Dumbbell Biceps Curl) is free weight exercise and some volunteers may not maintain their arm within a fixed space all the time. For exercise $E1$ (i.e., Barbell Bench Press), some volunteers easily perform too fast or too slow depending on the weights.

In addition, Fig. 6.10b presents the precision, recall and F_1 score for each exercise type, respectively. The average value of precision, recall and F_1 score of each exercise are all around 95%. Although the recall of exercise $E4$ (i.e., running) is 100%, we observe that it has the lowest precision among all 12 exercises, which indicates other exercises are more likely to be mistakenly classified as this exercise. This may be caused by the fact that arm swings are naturally moving in space and some volunteers freely perform some type of exercise too fast which also involve all axes sensor readings. The above results support that the proposed system can extract accurate information for exercise type recognition through wrist-worn smartwatch.

6.6.4 Workout Recognition Using Smartphone

We then evaluate workout recognition by using smartphone since arm-mounted phone have been widely used in people's daily exercise. We present the results from smartphone in Fig. 6.10c and d. Results show 91% average recognition accuracy for exercise recognition. We find exercise $E4$ still has the lowest precision which is consistent with the results collected from smartwatch since the volunteers wear smartwatch and smartphone on the same arm to make fair comparison.

Comparison Between Using Smartwatches and Using Smartphones Our system presents high accuracy of workout recognition for both smartphones and smartwatches. Comparing results between smartwatches and smartphones, we found that results obtained from smartwatches are better than results from smartphones. The average recognition accuracy of smartwatch is 95% whereas smartphones has a 91% average recognition accuracy. This observation is due to the fact that for exercise recognition, the space scope of the arm gesture trajectories was constrained by the machine for some exercise and most of the exercises require users to use their hands to grab and therefore the smartwatch on the wrist are close to hand and reflect more similar movement as machine or dumbbell.

6.6.5 Repetition Detection Accuracy

Finally, we evaluate the system by showing our detection accuracy for exercises. For workout exercise detection, the average detection accuracy reaches 99%. The

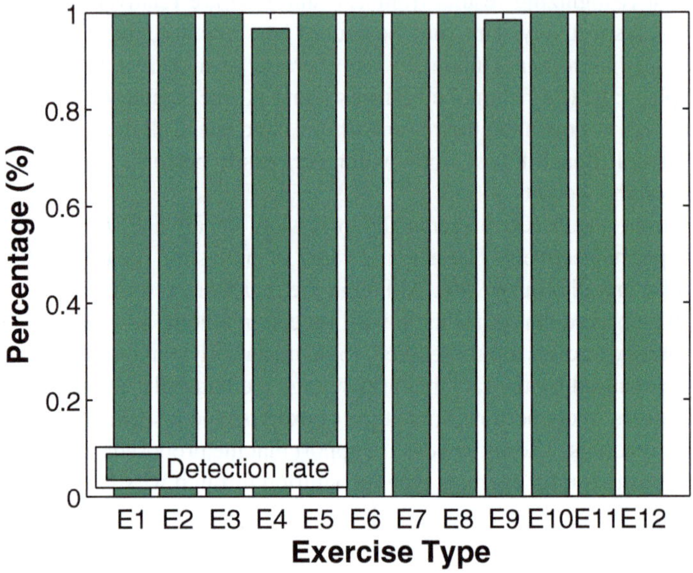

Fig. 6.11 Detection rate of exercise repetitions by using smartwatch

lowest detection accuracy occurs at running exercise $E4$ (i.e., step detection) on a treadmill but it still achieves around 95% detection accuracy as shown in Fig. 6.11. Such relative low detection accuracy of running exercise is due to occasionally holding on the handrails or wiping perspiration while running. The above results show that our system can accurately detect reps, and such high detection accuracy supports that fine-grained statistical information is reliable.

6.7 Summary

In this chapter, we propose an integrated mobile solution that can conduct systematic fitness monitoring and provide performance review based on a single off-the-shelf wearable device (e.g., wrist-worn wearables or arm-mounted smartphones). The proposed system has the capability to perform fine-grained exercise recognition including exercise types, the number of sets and repetitions by using inertial sensors from wearable devices without user involvement. Two novel metrics, exercise form score and workout review plane, are developed to provide effective review and recommendation for achieving effective workout and preventing injuries. To ensure the system accuracy and robustness, the system uses the earth/human coordinate system to align and integrate sensor readings from various device orientations. Extensive experiments involving 12 participants doing workout for over half a year time period demonstrate that the system successfully takes one step forward to provide the integrated fitness monitoring system with over 90% workout analysis accuracy. By integrating other existing sensors such as shoe sensors (https://secure-nikeplus.nike.com/plus/products/) and ankle-based belt, the system can be extended to monitor non-arm based exercises. In addition, our system can further reduce the energy consumption by utilizing location information. The system only needs to start sampling when detecting gym or fitness center nearby through the assistant of GPS and we left this part in our future work.

References

1. American College of Sports Medicine, et al.: ACSM's Guidelines for Exercise Testing and Prescription. Lippincott Williams & Wilkins, Philadelphia (2013)
2. Arney, J.: You should be in pictures! experts share tips on how to produce a quality fitness video for any purpose. IDEA Fitness J. **2**(1), 86–90 (2005)
3. Chang, K.H., Chen, M.Y., Canny, J.: Tracking free-weight exercises. In: Proceedings of the 9th International Conference on Ubiquitous Computing (ACM UbiComp) (2007)
4. Cheng, H.T., Sun, F.T., Griss, M., Davis, P., Li, J., You, D.: Nuactiv: recognizing unseen new activities using semantic attribute-based learning. In: Proceeding of the 11th Annual International Conference on Mobile Systems, Applications, and Services (ACM Mobisys) (2013)
5. Deller Jr., J.R., Proakis, J.G., Hansen, J.H.: Discrete Time Processing of Speech Signals, 1st edn. Prentice Hall PTR, Hoboken (1993)
6. Ding, H., Shangguan, L., Yang, Z., Han, J., Zhou, Z., Yang, P., Xi, W., Zhao, J.: Femo: A platform for free-weight exercise monitoring with rfids. In: Proceedings of the 13th ACM Conference on Embedded Networked Sensor Systems (ACM Sensys), pp. 141–154 (2015)
7. Hao, T., Xing, G., Zhou, G.: Runbuddy: a smartphone system for running rhythm monitoring. In: Proceedings of the 2015 ACM International Joint Conference on Pervasive and Ubiquitous Computing (ACM Ubicomp) (2015)
8. Lindberg, B.: On smoothing and extrapolation for the trapezoidal rule. BIT Numer. Math. **11**(1), 29–52 (1971)
9. Liu, J., Wang, Y., Chen, Y., Yang, J., Chen, X., Cheng, J.: Tracking vital signs during sleep leveraging off-the-shelf wifi. In: Proceedings of the 16th ACM International Symposium on Mobile Ad Hoc Networking and Computing (ACM Mobihoc), pp. 267–276 (2015)
10. Mifflin, M.D., St Jeor, S.T., Hill, L.A., Scott, B.J., Daugherty, S.A., Koh, Y.: A new predictive equation for resting energy expenditure in healthy individuals. Am. J. Clin. Nutr. **51**(2), 241–247 (1990)
11. Mokaya, F., Lucas, R., Noh, H.Y., Zhang, P.: Myovibe: vibration based wearable muscle activation detection in high mobility exercises. In: Proceedings of the 2015 ACM International Joint Conference on Pervasive and Ubiquitous Computing (ACM Ubicomp), pp. 27–38 (2015)
12. Parate, A., Chiu, M.C., Chadowitz, C., Ganesan, D., Kalogerakis, E.: RisQ: recognizing smoking gestures with inertial sensors on a wristband. In: Proceedings of the 12th Annual International Conference on Mobile Systems, Applications, and Services (ACM MobiSys), pp. 149–161 (2014)
13. Ren, Y., Chen, Y., Chuah, M.C., Yang, J.: Smartphone based user verification leveraging gait recognition for mobile healthcare systems. In: Proceedings of the 10th Annual IEEE Communications Society Conference on Sensor, Mesh and Ad Hoc Communications and Networks (IEEE SECON) (2013)
14. Ren, Z., Yuan, J., Meng, J., Zhang, Z.: Robust part-based hand gesture recognition using kinect sensor. IEEE Trans. Multimedia **15**(5), 1110–1120 (2013)

15. Thomaz, E., Essa, I., Abowd, G.D.: A practical approach for recognizing eating moments with wrist-mounted inertial sensing. In: Proceedings of the 2015 ACM International Joint Conference on Pervasive and Ubiquitous Computing (ACM Ubicomp), pp. 1029–1040 (2015)
16. Vapnik, V.N., Vapnik, V.: Statistical Learning Theory, vol. 1. Wiley, New York (1998)
17. Vlasic, D., Adelsberger, R., Vannucci, G., Barnwell, J., Gross, M., Matusik, W., Popović, J.: Practical motion capture in everyday surroundings. ACM Trans. Graph. **26**, 35 (2007)
18. Wang, Y., Liu, J., Chen, Y., Gruteser, M., Yang, J., Liu, H.: E-eyes: device-free location-oriented activity identification using fine-grained wifi signatures. In: Proceedings of the 20th Annual International Conference on Mobile Computing and Networking (ACM Mobicom), pp. 617–628 (2014)

Chapter 7
Fine-grained Gesture Recognition and Sign Language Interpretation via Photoplethysmography (PPG) on Smartwatches

In addition to the application of inertial sensors in wearable devices, various other sensors have been utilized to broaden the scope of sensing applications. This chapter challenges the conventional perception of Photoplethysmography (PPG) and paves the way for innovative use of PPG in commercially available wearable technology. It pays special attention to its potential in the field of human-computer interaction, specifically in enabling fine-grained gesture recognition. We demonstrate that it is possible to leverage the widely deployed PPG sensors in wrist-worn wearable devices to enable finger-level gesture recognition, which could facilitate many emerging human-computer interactions (e.g., sign-language interpretation and virtual reality). While prior solutions in gesture recognition require dedicated devices (e.g., video cameras or IR sensors) or leverage various signals in the environments (e.g., sound, RF or ambient light), this chapter introduces the first PPG-based gesture recognition system that can differentiate fine-grained hand gestures at finger level using commodity wearables. Our innovative system harnesses the unique blood flow changes in a user's wrist area to distinguish the user's finger and hand movements. The insight is that hand gestures involve a series of muscle and tendon movements that compress the arterial geometry with different degrees, resulting in significant motion artifacts to the blood flow with different intensity and time duration. By leveraging the unique characteristics of the motion artifacts to PPG, our system can accurately extract the gesture-related signals from the significant background noise (i.e., pulses), and identify different minute finger-level gestures. Extensive experiments are conducted with over 3600 gestures collected from 10 adults. Our prototype study using two commodity PPG sensors can differentiate nine finger-level gestures from American Sign Language with an average recognition accuracy over 88%, suggesting that our PPG-based finger-level gesture recognition system is promising to be one of the most critical components in sign language translation using wearables. The structure of the remainder of this chapter is as follows: Sect. 7.1 begins by providing the research background. This is followed by Sect. 7.2, in which we review the current literature in the field. Subsequently,

X. Guo et al., *Mobile Technologies for Smart Healthcare System Design*,
Wireless Networks, https://doi.org/10.1007/978-3-031-57345-3_7

in Sect. 7.3, we delve into the principles of gesture recognition employing PPG sensors, demonstrating the potential for finger-level gesture recognition using these sensors. In Sect. 7.4, we address the challenges encountered during system implementation and offer comprehensive details on system design. Section 7.5 furnishes a thorough depiction of the system's implementation. Section 7.6 encompasses the system's evaluation. Lastly, Sect. 7.7 encapsulates the chapter with a succinct summary.

7.1 Background

The popularity of wrist-worn wearable devices has a sharp increase since 2015, an estimation of 101.4 million wrist-worn wearable devices will be shipped worldwide in 2019 [13]. Such increasing popularity of wrist-worn wearables creates a unique opportunity of using various sensing modalities in wearables for pervasive hand or finger gesture recognition. Hand and finger gestures usually have a diverse combinations and thus present rich information that can facilitate many complicated human computer interaction (HCI) applications, for example wearable controls, virtual reality (VR)/augmented reality (AR), and automatic sign language translation. Taking the automatic sign language translation as an example illustrated in Fig. 7.1, a wrist-worn wearable device (e.g., a smartwatch or a wristband) could leverage its sensors to realize and convert sign language into audio and text and back again, which will greatly help people who are deaf or have difficulty hearing to communicate with those who do not know the sign language.

Existing solutions of gesture recognition mainly rely on cameras [14, 17, 21] microphones [16, 18], radio frequency (RF) [5, 20, 23] or special body sensors (e.g., Electromyography (SEMG) [15], Electrical Impedance Tomography (EIT) sensor [30], and electrocardiogram (ECG) sensor [29]). The approaches using cameras face occlusion and privacy issues. Microphones are vulnerable to ambient acoustic noises. The RF-based approaches are usually known to be device-free, but they are very sensitive to indoor multipath effects or RF interference. Using special body sensors for gesture recognition is more robust to environmental noises but requires extra cost and manpower of installation. Recently, motion sensors in wearables present their great potential in hand and finger gesture recognition on the wrist [27, 28], but motion sensors are sensitive to body motions and are thus difficult to identify fine-grained finger-level gestures, such as sign language gestures.

In this work, we propose to recognize the fine-grained finger-level gestures such as sign language using low-cost PPG sensors in wearable devices. We study the unique PPG features resulted from finger-level gestures, and carefully devise a system that can effectively detect, segment, extract, and classify finger-level gestures based on only PPG measurements. The basic idea of our system is examining the blood flow changes resulted from finger-level gestures based on the PPG measurements, which are collected by low-cost PPG sensors in wrist-worn wearable devices. The advantages of our approach are twofold. First, our system could be

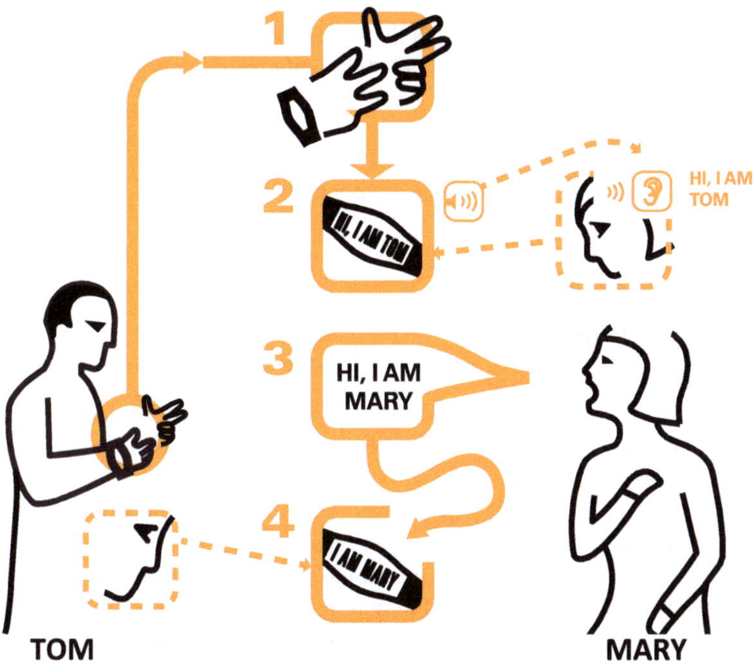

Fig. 7.1 Illustration of the automatic sign language translation using wearables in daily communications

easily applied to billions of existing wrist-worn wearable devices without extra cost, enabling every wrist-worn wearable device to recognize fine-grained gestures on users' fingers (e.g., sign language). Second, our system only relies on wrist-worn PPG sensors, which directly obtain gesture related features without the impact of environmental changes (e.g., ambient light, sound, RF) and moderate body movements (e.g., walking, turning body, slow arm movements), thus is more robust in practical scenarios.

In this study, we demonstrate the potential of utilizing PPG sensors found in wrist-worn wearable devices to recognize fine-grained finger-level gestures. Through the development of a machine-learning approach, we leverage the distinctive gesture-related PPG patterns captured by these wearables on the wrist, marking the first work of its kind in recognizing such gestures using readily available commodity PPG sensors. By exploring the physical meaning and characteristics of PPG measurements collected from the wrist sensor, we devise a novel data extraction method that effectively separates minute finger movement-induced PPG measurements from the continuous background noise caused by human pulses. Furthermore, we establish the feasibility of accurately identifying intricate finger-level gestures with subtle variations, such as those found in sign language, by exploiting a range of features extracted from the unique gesture-related PPG patterns in different signal spaces, including dynamic time warping, wavelet transform, and Fourier transform. To validate our approach, we conduct experiments involving ten participants who wear our prototype comprising two off-the-shelf PPG sensors and an Arduino board. The results showcase an impressive average accuracy of over 88% in identifying nine finger-level gestures from American Sign Language. These findings highlight the promising potential of our PPG-based finger-level gesture recognition system as a crucial component in sign language translation using wearable devices.

7.2 Related Work

In general, current techniques for gesture recognition can be broadly categorized into four categories (i.e., vision-based, RF-based, acoustic-based and body sensor based) as follows:

A couple of vision-based approaches have been developed to recognize hand/body gestures with the help of cameras (e.g., Microsoft Kinect [21] and leap motion [17]) or visible light (e.g., LiSense [14]). However, these approaches are sensitive to the ambient light and may require users to have the line of sight to the cameras or need specific light sensing equipment installation.

RF-based approaches have become increasingly important due to the prevalent wireless environments. For instance, WiDraw [23] and Wisee [20] propose to use channel state information(CSI) and Doppler shifts of wireless signals to achieve fine-grained gesture recognition, respectively. WiTrack [1] and WiTrack2.0 [2] can track multiple users by examining the multi-path effects of Frequency-Modulated Continuous-Wave (FMCW) signals. These approaches, however, either can be easily affected by environmental changes such as people walking or require dedicated and costly devices such as the Universal Software Radio Peripheral (USRP).

Acoustic-based approaches are also explored by several studies. For instance, CAT [16] and FingerIO [18] track a smartphone's motion and a finger's dynamics by using audio components (e.g., multiple external speakers, device's microphones), respectively. However, these approaches need occupy device's speaker/microphone and external audio hardware (e.g., nearby speakers), which is not always available in many real-world scenarios.

In addition, several customized wearable devices, which can be worn on users' forearm or wrist, are designed to capture the hand gesture by capturing either Surface Electromyography (SEMG) signals [15], Electrical Impedance Tomography (EIT) [30] or electrocardiogram (ECG) [29]. However, these solutions need extra hardware supports and are not compatible with existing mobile/wearable devices. Another body of related work is using motion sensors in wrist-worn wearables to achieve hand and finger gesture recognition [27, 28]. The solution, however, is sensitive to body/arm motions and cannot identify fine-grained finger-level gestures, such as sign language gestures.

Different from previous work, in this chapter, we propose to innovatively use the photoplethysmogram (PPG) sensor, which is originally used for heart rate detection in the most of the commodity wearable devices (e.g., smartwatch and wristband), to perform fine-grained finger-level gesture recognition and detection. To the best of our knowledge, it is the first wrist-worn PPG sensor based gesture recognition system. With the proposed scheme, we envision that most wearable device manufacturers would open the interface of PPG raw readings to developers soon.

7.3 PPG Preliminaries and Feasibility Study

7.3.1 Background of Wearable PPG Sensors

During the past few years, more and more commodity wrist-worn wearables (e.g., smartwaches and activity trackers) are equipped with Photoplethysmography (PPG) sensors on their back as illustrated in Fig. 7.2. These wrist-worn PPG sensors are mainly designed to measure and record users' heart rates. Specifically, a typical PPG sensor consists of a couple of LEDs and a photodiode/photodetector (PD), which detects the light reflected from the wrist tissue. The principle of PPG is the detection of blood volume changes in the microvascular bed of tissue. When light travels through biological tissue, different substances (e.g., skin, blood and blood vessel, tendon, and bone) have the different absorptivities of light. Usually, blood absorbs more light than the surrounding tissue. Therefore, by utilizing a PD to capture the intensity changes of the light reflected from the tissue, the wearable device can derive the blood flow changes in the wrist-area tissue and calculate the pulse rate or even blood pressure [4].

It is important to note that most PPG sensors embedded in commodity wearable devices use green LEDs as light source has much greater absorptivity for oxyhemoglobin and deoxyhemoglobin compared to other light sources (e.g., red or infrared light) [25]. We thus use green-LED PPG sensors in this work to study and evaluate PPG based gesture recognition.

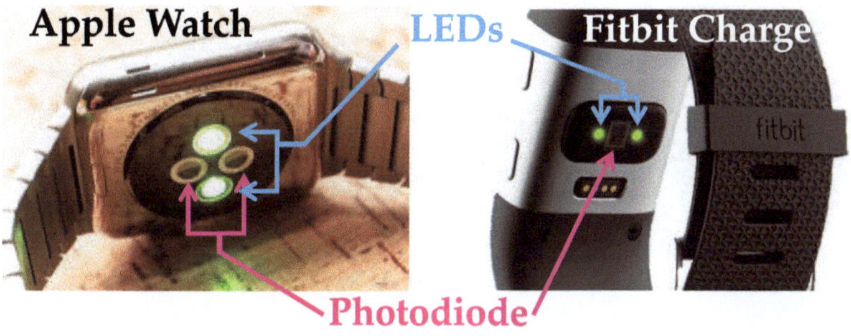

Fig. 7.2 Example of PPG sensors in wrist-worn wearable devices

7.3.2 Gesture Recognition Using PPG Sensors

The current use of PPG in wearables is limited to heart rate, pulse oximetry and blood pressure monitoring. Such applications only focus on examining regular blood flow changing patterns in the radial artery and the ulnar artery, and consider mechanical movement artifacts as noise [25]. In this work, we put forward an innovative idea of using readily available PPG in wearables for finger-level gesture recognition. We show that hand gestures, especially finger gestures (i.e., flexion, extension, abduction, and adduction), result in significant motion artifacts to PPG. The reason behind this is that the two major muscles controlling hand gestures [12], namely flexor digitorum superficialis and flexor hallucis longus, are right beside the radial artery and the ulnar artery as illustrated in Fig. 7.3. Any hand or finger gestures would involve a series of complicated muscle and tendon movements that may compress the arterial geometry with different degrees. Since the blood absorbs most of the green light, the changes of the light reflected from the wrist area present different degrees of disturbances of the flood flow in terms of the shapes and duration of PPG waveforms. Current PPG sensors in off-the-shelf wearables are usually equipped with two green LED and photodiodes to ensure accurate pulse estimation by increasing the diversity (i.e., monitoring blood flow changes at different locations on the wrist). In this work, we mimic this approach and utilize two separated PPG sensors at close but different locations on the wrist to ensure our gesture recognition accuracy.

7.3.3 Feasibility Study

In order to explore the feasibility of using PPG sensors in commodity wearables for finger-level gesture recognition, we conduct five sets of experiments on a sensing platform prototyped with two off-the-shelf PPG sensors (i.e., a photodiode sensor

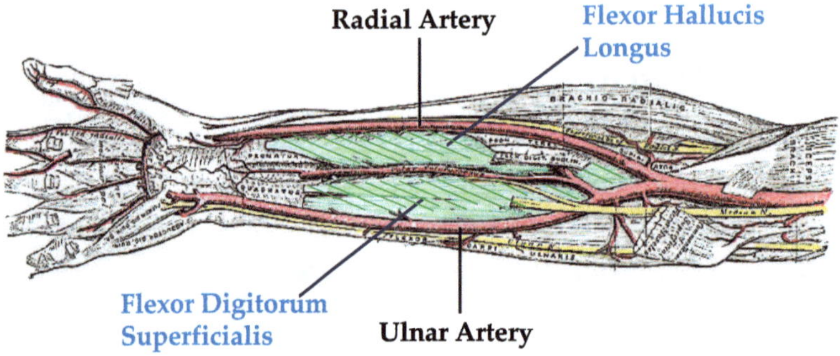

Fig. 7.3 Illustration of the finger movement related muscles in the anatomy of a human forearm

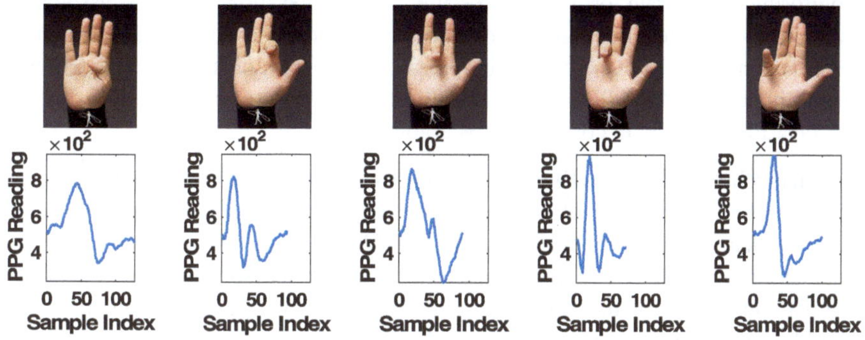

Fig. 7.4 Example of PPG readings associated with five finger-bending gestures in the feasibility study

and a green LED) connecting to an Arduino UNO (Rev3) board, which continuously collects PPG readings at 100 Hz and save them to a PC. During the experiments, a user wears a wristband to fix two off-the-shelf PPG sensors on the inner side of the wrist, and respectively bends each of his fingers as illustrated in Fig. 7.4 to emulate the simplest elements of sign language gestures. Specifically, in each set of the experiments, the user bends one of his finger 10 times with 8s between each bending. We record the process of the experiments using a video camera synchronized with the PPG measurements to determine the starting and ending time of each finger bending gesture.

We extract the PPG sensor readings within the time window between the starting and ending points identified in the video footage of each gesture and examine their changing patterns. As we expected, bending different fingers result in different unique patterns in PPG readings. Figure 7.4 presents an example of the unique patterns in PPG that correspond to bending different fingers, which is from one out of the two sensors. Moreover, we notice that same finger movements generate similar patterns, which demonstrates that it is possible to utilize readily available PPG sensors in wearables for fine-grained gesture recognition.

7.4 System Challenges and System Design

7.4.1 Challenges

In order to build a system that can recognize fine-grained finger-level gestures (e.g., sign language) using PPG sensors in wearable devices, a number of challenges need to be addressed.

Re-using the PPG Sensors in Wearables for Finger-level Gesture Recognition The PPG sensors in commodity wearable devices are specifically designed for monitoring pulse rate or blood pressure. The blood flow changes associated with finger-level gestures have much shorter duration and do not have repetitive patterns compared to those caused by pulses. Our system thus needs to detect and discriminate the unique PPG patterns of different finger movements by re-using the low-cost PPG sensors in commodity wearable devices.

Gesture-related PPG Readings Interfered by Pulses In this work, PPG readings corresponding to finger-level gestures are treated as target signals that our system wants to identify and examine. Therefore, the PPG readings resulted from pulses are considered to be the noise. Such noise always exists and sometimes has intensity comparable to that of the signals caused by finger-level gestures. Our approach should be intelligent enough to separate relevant useful signals from the complicated noise caused by pulses.

Accurate Finger Gesture Recognition Using Single Sensing Modality on the Wrist It is also challenging to achieve high accuracy in fine-grained finger-level gesture recognition by using the readily available but coarse-grained wrist-worn PPG technique. Commodity wearable devices usually only have few PPG sensors that are placed very close to each other. Such layout limits the coverage of the PPG sensors on the wrist and the diversity of sensor readings, which could significantly impact the performance of gesture recognition. We thus need to explore the critical features of PPG readings in different domains to achieve accurate finger-level gesture recognition.

7.4.2 PPG-based Gesture Recognition Sensing System Design

The basic idea of our system is examining the blood flow changes collected by readily available PPG sensors in commodity wrist-worn wearable devices to differentiate different fine-grained finger-level gestures. Toward this end, we design a machine-learning approach that mainly contains two major steps: *Training Phase* and *Classification Phase*. As illustrated in Fig. 7.5, our system first takes as inputs the PPG measurements from wrist-worn PPG sensors. Then it conducts *Coarse-grained Gesture Detection and Reference Sensor Determination* to determine whether there is any gesture being performed based on the signal energy after mitigating the noise from pulses. Then the system automatically determines the *Reference Sensor*, which is the sensor presenting significant (i.e. containing more energy) gesture-related PPG patterns compared to those related to pulses. The system will keep monitoring the PPG sensor if there is no gesture detected. Otherwise, it will further process the raw PPG measurements depending on whether it is in the *Training Phase* or *Classification Phase*.

Training Phase In the *Training Phase*, we collect labeled PPG measurements for each gesture and build binary classifiers for each user. Specifically, we perform *Fine-grained PPG Data Segmentation Using Energy and DTW* to accurately extract

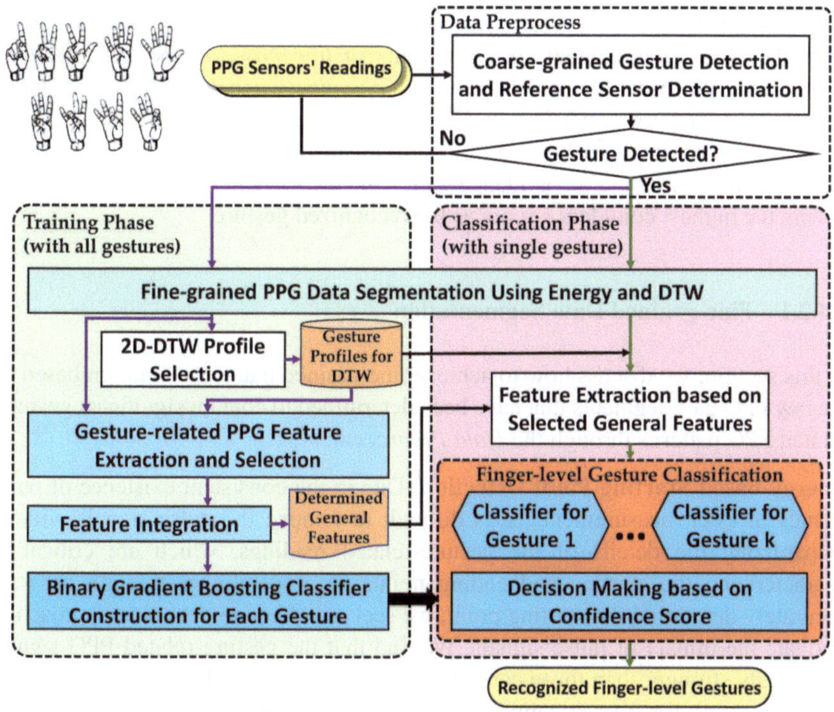

Fig. 7.5 Overview of the PPG-based finger-level gesture recognition system

the segments containing gesture-related PPG measurements between the estimated starting and ending points of gestures, which are obtained by examining the energy and dynamic time warping (DTW) distance to pulse profiles in a sliding window.

After segmentation, our system calculates the 2D-DTW distances between every two segments for every gesture in *2D-DTW Profile Selection* and selects three profile segments that are most representative for each gesture (i.e., having the minimum average 2D-DTW distance to other segments of the same gesture). The selected profile segments will be used to calculate the DTW features in the *Classification Phase*. Meanwhile, the system performs *PPG Feature Extraction and Selection* to derive a variety of features in different signal spaces (e.g., discrete wavelet transform, fast Fourier transform) and selects the critical features that can effectively capture the unique gesture-related PPG patterns for each gesture. Because the selected critical feature sets are optimized for each gesture, the system further derives a super set of the selected critical features in *Feature Integration* to ensure the system performance. Next, we perform *Binary Gradient Boosting Classifier Construction for Each Gesture* to train a binary classifier for each target gesture using Gradient Boosting.

Classification Phase In the *Classification Phase*, our system collects testing PPG measurements in real time and determines which finger gesture has been performed based on the classification results. The system extracts the selected critical features from the PPG data segments in *Feature Extraction based on Selected General Features* and performs *Finger-level Gesture Classification* to determine which target gesture has been performed. Specifically, the system processes the extracted features using the binary gradient boosting classifiers built for target gestures in parallel. Each classifier generates a confidence score, and the system takes the target gesture having the highest confidence score as the recognized gesture.

7.4.2.1 Fine-grained Data Segmentation

In this section, we discuss how to achieve fine-grained data segmentation based on the raw PPG data segments that have been determined to contain significant gesture-related PPG patterns through the *Data Preprocess*.

Energy-based Starting Point Detection Due to the consistent existence of pulse signals in PPG measurements, it is difficult to remove the pulse signals without jeopardizing the details of the gesture-related readings, which are critical to characterizing the starting and ending points of a specific gesture. In order to accurately determine the starting point, we seek an effective detection approach to mitigate the impact of pulse signals. We find that the gesture-related PPG signals are usually stronger than those caused by pulses as illustrated in Fig. 7.6a, because gestures usually involve dynamics of major forearm muscles/tendons close to the sensor on the wrist. Inspired by the above observation, we design an energy-based starting point detection scheme to effectively estimate the starting of gesture-related PPG signals without removing the interference of pulses.

The basic idea of our energy-based starting point detection method is to determine the time corresponding to the local maximum of the short-time energy of PPG signals. The reason behind this is that when using a sliding window with the same length of a signal to calculate the short-time energy of the signal, the energy reaches its maximum value when the signal entirely falls into the window. Therefore, by carefully choosing the size of the sliding window (e.g., the average length of target gesture-related signals), the starting point of the gesture-related signals would be the same time when the short-time energy of the signals reaches its maximum. In particular, given the data segment containing gesture-related PPG signals $P(t)$ from the *Coarse-grained Gesture Segmentation*, the starting point detection problem can be formulated as the following objective function:

$$\arg\max_{\tau} \ (P(\tau) - \mathbf{1}\theta)P(\tau)^T, \tag{7.1}$$

where $P(\tau) = [p(\tau), p(\tau + \delta) \cdots, p(\tau + W)]$, $p(\tau)$ denotes the amplitude of the PPG signal at time τ, δ represents the PPG sensor sampling interval, W is the length of the sliding window, θ is the threshold used to avoid finding the local maximum energy resulted from pulse signals, $\mathbf{1}$ is an all-one vector of the same length as $P(\tau)$, and T indicates the transpose operation. The above problem can be easily

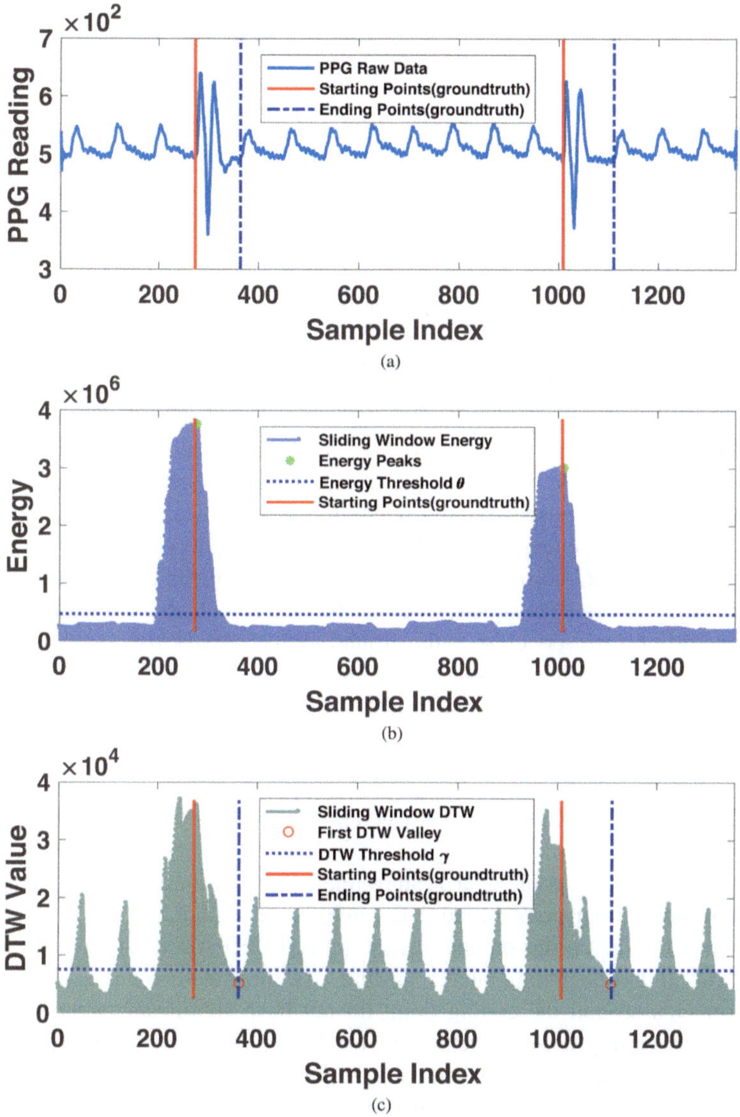

Fig. 7.6 Example of detecting starting and ending point of a gesture-related PPG measurements using energy and DTW. (**a**) PPG raw data with gesture ground truth (**b**) Short-time energy of PPG (**c**) Short-time DTW distance to pulse profile

solved through simple 1-D searching within the period derived from coarse-grained gesture segmentation.

Through our preliminary study on the time length of 1080 finger gestures performed by three users as shown in Fig. 7.7, we find that the length of gesture-related signals has the range between 0.7 and 1.4 s with an average of 1.2 s.

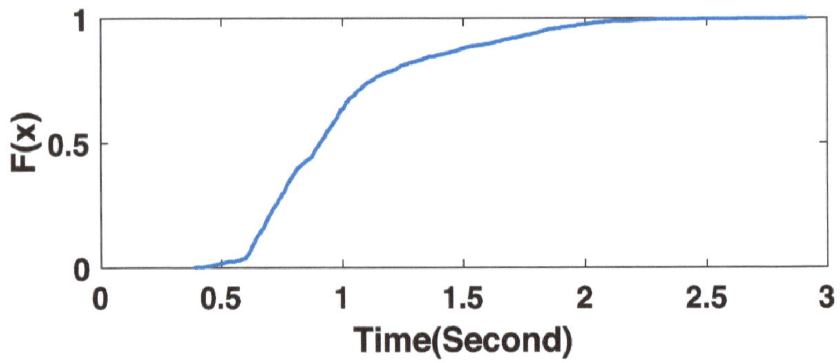

Fig. 7.7 Preliminary study: CDF of the duration of 1080 gestures from 3 users

Therefore, we empirically determine the length of the sliding window as 1.2 s to ensure the accuracy of our energy-based starting point detection. Note that the threshold θ is user-specific and needs to be dynamically determined by the maximum short-time energy of the PPG signals when there is no gesture detected in the *Coarse-grained Gesture Detection*. Figure 7.6b illustrates the short-time energy corresponding to the PPG signals in Fig. 7.6a. We can clearly see that the energy peaks in Fig. 7.6b are very close to the ground truth observed from the synchronized video footage, suggesting that our algorithm could promisingly capture the starting point of gestures in the PPG measurements.

7.4.2.2 DTW-based Ending Point Detection

Detecting the ending point of a gesture-related signal is more challenging than detecting the starting point because the muscles are more relaxed at the end of the gesture and the corresponding gesture-related PPG signals are usually weaker than those at the beginning of the gesture. As illustrated in Fig. 7.6a, the PPG measurements around the ending point do not have significant patterns that can facilitate the ending point detection. However, we find that gesture-related PPG signals are usually immediately followed by pulse signals, which are very clear and easy to identify. Hence, instead of directly locating the ending point based on PPG readings, we design a DTW-based ending point detection scheme, which aims to identify the starting time of the first pulse signal following the gesture-related signal. We employ the dynamic time warping (DTW) to measure the similarity between the user's pulse profile P_{pulse} and the PPG measurements collected after the already-detected starting point of the gesture.

Intuitively, the time when the DTW value reaches the minimum is the starting time of the pulse signals and also the ending point of the gesture-related signals. We adopt DTW because it can stretch and compress parts of PPG measurements to accommodate the small variations in the pulse signals. To summary up, this ending point detection problem is defined as follows:

$$\arg\min_{t} \; DTW(P(t), P_{pulse}), \quad s.t., \tau < t \leq \tau + W_p, \tag{7.2}$$

where $DTW(\cdot, \cdot)$ is the function to calculate the DTW distance, $P(t)$ has the same definition as $P(\tau)$ in Eq. (7.1), W_p is the time duration for the gesture, and τ is the detected starting point. After searching the DTW distances for all $P(t)$, we find the time index of the first local minimum in the DTW distances (i.e., the starting time of the first pulse after the gesture) as the ending point of the gesture-related signals. Figure 7.6c presents the DTW between a selected pulse profile and the raw PPG measurements in Fig. 7.6a with $W_p = 0.88$ s. From the figure, we can observe that the time indexes of the detected first local minimum DTW values are very close to the ground truth of the ending time of the two gestures, which demonstrates the effectiveness of the DTW-based ending point detection scheme.

The pulse profile P_{pulse} can be extracted from the PPG measurements that are collected when there is no gesture performed (e.g., at the beginning of the training phase). In particular, we first detect the pulse signal peaks in the PPG measurements. Given the fact that a typical PPG pulse signal always has a peak, if the pulse signal peak is located at t_p, so the PPG measurements between $[t_p - t_d, t_p + t_s]$ are identified as the user's pulse profile. In this work, we respectively choose $t_d = 0.2$ s and $t_s = 0.6$ s based on the duration of diastole (i.e., $0.15 \sim 0.26$ s) and systole (i.e., $0.44 \sim 0.74$ s) phases of the vascular system reflected in a typical PPG pulse signal [7], which can effectively extract all users' pulse profile.

7.4.2.3 Segmentation on Inconspicuous Gesture-related Patterns

Our DTW-based ending point detection can accurately determine the ending point if the gesture-related PPG pattern has significant amplitudes compared to those of the pulse-related patterns. However, in rare cases, the gesture-related PPG patterns may not have significant amplitudes when the sensor is at the locations far away from the arteries. Note that such inconspicuous patterns are not easy to be extracted as their boundaries with pulse-related patterns are very vague, but they still contain rich information that could greatly facilitate gesture recognition. In this work, we find that when using two PPG sensors close to each other on the wrist, at least one of the sensors can generate gesture-related PPG patterns with significant amplitudes. Inspired by this observation, we adopt a reference-based approach to accurately determine the ending point for the inconspicuous gesture-related PPG patterns.

In particular, assuming our system identifies the ending point t_R on the sensor R with significant gesture-related PPG patterns (i.e., *Reference Sensor*) using our DTW-based method, the system further derives the ending point at the other sensor D as $t_D = t_R + \Delta T$, where ΔT is the time delay of the ending point on sensor R. According to our empirical study, ΔT is nonzero and stable between two sensors across different gestures. Since muscles and tendons at different locations of the forearm compress the arteries with different pressure and duration when performing a gesture, the gesture-related patterns captured by the PPG sensors at different locations will last different time periods. Because the system can always find multiple gestures that generate significant PPG patterns on both sensors, ΔT can be easily estimated in the *Training Phase* by calculating the average time difference of the ending points from the gestures where both sensors are determined to be *Reference Sensors*.

7.4.3 Sign Language Gesture Classification

In this part, we explore the PPG features that could facilitate gesture recognition and discuss how to build the binary classifier using Gradient Boosting and perform gesture classification in the *Training Phase* and *Classification Phase*.

7.4.3.1 PPG Feature Extraction and Selection

To capture the characteristics of unique gesture-related PPG patterns, we explore the efficacy of different kinds of features including typical temporal statistics (e.g., mean, variance, standard deviation (STD)), cross-correlation, autoregressive (AR), dynamic time warping (DTW), fast Fourier transform (FFT), discrete wavelet transform (DWT), and Wigner Ville distribution as listed in Table 7.1. The features can be categorized into three types: *Time Domain*, *Frequency Domain*, and *Time-Frequency Domain*, which are designed to capture the detailed characteristics of the gesture-related PPG patterns across different frequency and time resolutions. While the *AR Coefficients*, *FFT*, *DWT*, *WVD*, and most of the *Classic Statistics* are all focusing on analyzing an individual sensor's measurements, the *Cross Correlation* and *2D-DTW* are promising for characterizing the unique gesture-based PPG patterns in terms of the relationship between a pair of sensors. Moreover, our *Time-Frequency (TF) Domain* features include three major TF types (i.e., non-parametric linear TF analysis (DWT), non-parametric quadratic TF analysis (WVD), and parametric time-varying based metric (AR)), which can well capture the dynamics of gestures in PPG measurements. In total, we extract 54 different features from each PPG sensor. Note that in order to calculate the 2D-DTW feature, our system first performs *2D-DTW Profile Selection* in the *Training Phase*, which calculates the 2D-DTW distance between every two segments for every gesture in the training data and selects three segments that have the minimum average 2D-DTW distance to other segments of the same gesture as the profile for later use in the *Classification Phase*.

Our system further employs the elastic net feature selection method [19] in the *Training Phase* to automatically choose the most discriminative ones from our extracted features. In particular, the system respectively performs the elastic net feature selection on the PPG features corresponding to every target gesture. Based on the one-stand-deviation rule [9], our system keeps the most significant highly

Table 7.1 List of extracted features

Category	Features (# of features)	Description
Time domain	Classic statistics (4): mean, peak-to-peak, RMS, variance	Descriptive statistics of each segment, reflecting the statistical characteristics of the unique gesture-related patterns.
	Cross correlation between sensors (9)	A vector of cross correlation coefficients between the segments from two PPG sensors based on a sequence of the lag values, characterizing the relationship between two PPG sensors in a gesture.
	2D-DTW to gesture profiles (9)	Similarity between PPG measurements from two sensors (i.e., 2D) and the corresponding g esture profiles, directly capturing the temporal shape characteristics of the unique gesture-related patterns.
Frequency domain	Fast fourier transform (< 5 Hz) (6): skewness, kurtosis, mean, median, var, peak-to-peak	Statistics of frequency components in the specific low frequency band, analyzing the unique PPG patterns in frequency domain.
Time-frequency domain	Discrete wavelet transform (4): mean, peak-to-peak, RMS, variance	Statistics of the third level decomposition of the wavelet transform using the Harr wavelet, revealing the details of gesture-related patterns at interested time and frequency scale.
	Wigner Ville distribution [8] (13): first-order derivative, frequency and time when the signal reaches the maximum, maximum energy (E^i_{max}) / minimum energy (E^i_{min}), differential energy ($E^i_{max} - E^i_{min}$), STD^i and AV^i of the energy within the ith sliding window	Fine-grained time-frequency features with high resolutions, capturing details of gesture-related patterns having short time duration.
	Autoregressive coefficients [26] (9)	Time variant coefficients that can capture the characteristics of gesture-related patterns independent of the patterns' time scales.

correlated features and eliminates noisy and redundant features to shrink the feature set and avoid overfitting. Next, in order to generalize the features set for classifying all target gestures, our system integrates the features selected for each target gesture and generates a general feature set $\mathbb{F}$ as follows:

$$\mathbb{F} = F(g_1) \cup \ldots \cup F(g_n), \tag{7.3}$$

where $F(g_n)$ is the selected feature set of the n_{th} target gesture g_n. After the feature selection and integration, we keep 46 *Determined General Features* in $\mathbb{F}$, which will be used in the *Classification Phase*. Figure 7.8 illustrates that our features

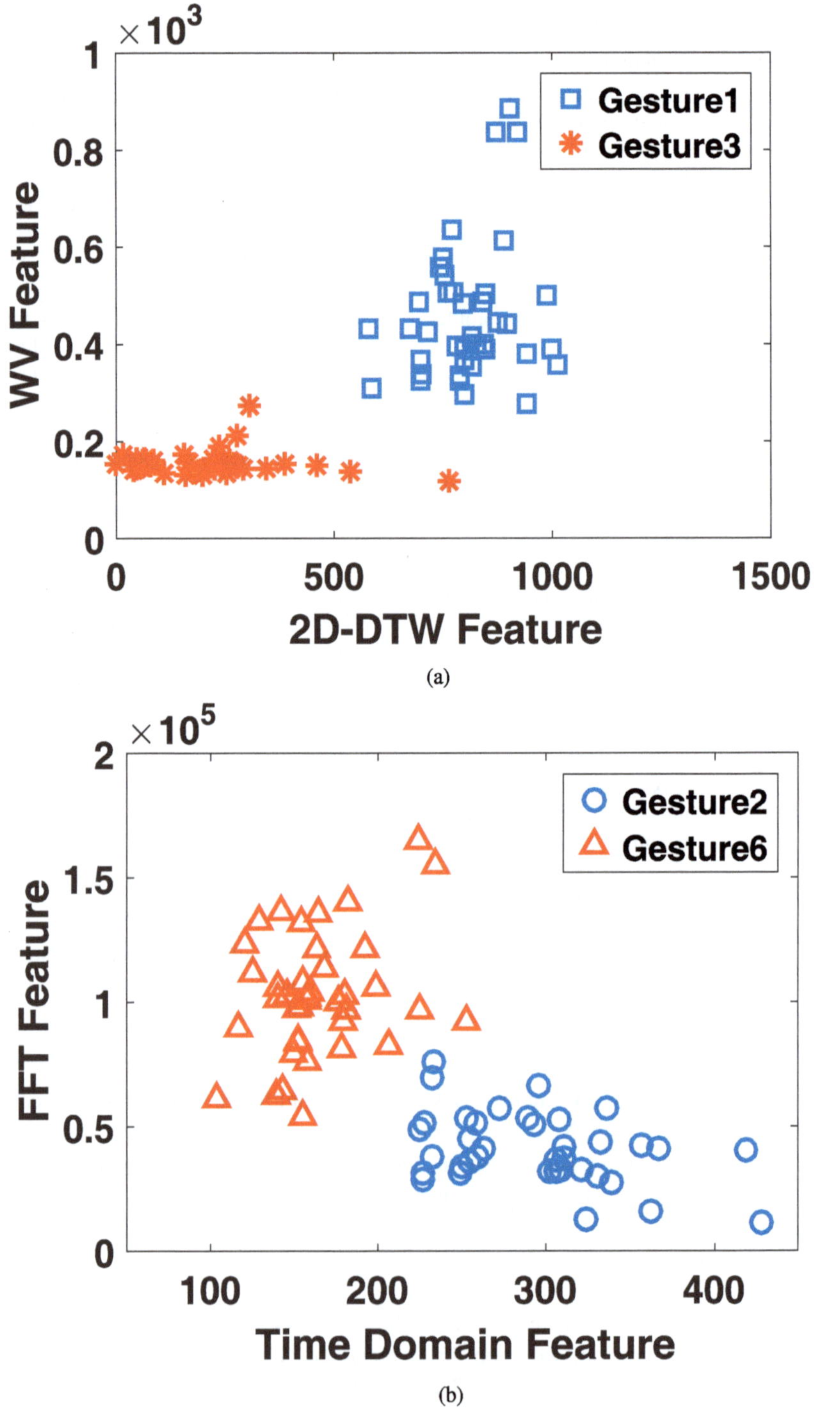

Fig. 7.8 Example of different finger-level gestures and corresponding features. (**a**) Gesture 1 and gesture 3 (**b**) Gesture 2 and gesture 6

can effectively capture different characteristics of PPG patterns for distinguishing different gestures.

7.4.3.2 Gradient Boosting Tree Based Classification

Next, we build a binary classifier for each target gesture by using the Gradient Boosting Tree (GBT). We choose GBT mainly because (1) GBT is famous for its robustness to various types of features with different scales, which is the exact case in our project (e.g., the mean value of the PPG signal reading of the gesture period is around 500, and the autoregressive coefficients are the numbers fluctuated around 0 with value less than (1). (2) GBT classifier is robust to the collinearity of feature data. Because our features are heterogeneous across different domains, it may result in unexpected correlation or unbalance ranges that possess the collinearity. Therefore, GBT would eliminate the efforts to normalize or whiten the feature data before classification [11]. We note that among all the machine learning methods, such as Random Forest (RF) and Support Vector Machine (SVM), adopted for our classifier implementation, GBT has the best performance.

Given N training samples $\{(x_i, y_i)\}$, where x_i and y_i represent the gesture-related feature set and corresponding label with respect to one specific gesture (i.e., $y_i = 1$ or -1 represents whether x_i is from this gesture), GBT seeks a function $\phi(x_i) = \sum_{m=1}^{M} \omega_m h_m(x_i)$ to iteratively select weak learners $h_j(\cdot)$ and their weights ω_j to minimize a loss function as follows:

$$\mathbf{L} = \sum_{i=1}^{N} L(y_i, \phi x_i). \tag{7.4}$$

Specifically, we adopt the GBT implementation from the library of SQBlib [6] for gesture-related feature training. Specifically, the loss function $L(\cdot)$ is chosen as the exponential loss $L = e^{-y_i \phi(x_i)}$ that applies enough shrinkage (i.e., 0.1) and number of iterations (i.e., $M = 2000$), and the sub-sampling of the training dataset is a fraction of 0.5. The above parameters adopted in GBT are optimized in terms of the speed and accuracy based on our empirical study. Once the loss function is determined, we next will build a binary gradient classifier $b_k(\cdots)$ for each profiled gesture $g_k, k = 1, \cdots, K$ to complete the *Training Phase*, and each binary gradient classifier will output a score for the testing feature set. The reason of using binary classifier is that binary classifier has high accuracy with distinguishing one gesture from other gestures, whereas a multi-classifier has relative lower accuracy when performs the same classification task [10].

In *Classification Phase*, our system uses the binary classifiers for all the gestures in parallel to classify previously unseen gesture-related feature set x. Specifically, we sum the stage score [24] of each binary classifier, and choose the label k of binary classifier $b_k(x)$ with highest score as the final classification.

7.5 System Implementation

Coarse-grained Gesture Detection and Segmentation To facilitate the fine-grained data extraction, our system preprocesses the raw PPG measurements to (1) determine whether there is a gesture performed or not based on the short-time energy of the PPG measurements; (2) and extract the PPG measurements that surely include the whole gesture-related PPG pattern. Specifically, the system first applies a high-pass filter to the raw PPG measurements to mitigate the interference of pulses. The reason to use the high-pass filter is that the finger-level gestures have more high-frequency components compared to the pulses, which are usually under 2 Hz [3]. In this work, we build a Butterworth high-pass filter with the cut-off frequency at 2 Hz. Note that we only use the filtering technique in the coarse-grained gesture detection, because the filter removes the low-frequency components of both pulse and gesture-related signals, which negatively impact the gesture recognition accuracy. Then the system decides whether there is a gesture performed or not depending on if the short-time energy of the filtered PPG measurements crosses a threshold τ or not. We set the threshold to $\tau = \mu + 3\delta$, where μ and δ are the mean and standard deviation of the short-time energy of the filtered PPG measurements collected during the time when the user is asked to be static (i.e., at the beginning of the training phase). When the system detects a gesture at t_g, we employ a fixed time window W_c to extract the raw PPG measurements within $[t_g, t_g + W_c]$ for the fine-grained segmentation. We set $W_c = 4.5$ s to ensure the window can cover all possible duration of gestures that we have observed in our preliminary study as shown in Fig. 7.7.

Reference Sensor Determination Intuitively, significant gesture-related PPG patterns could result in accurate data segmentation. However, we notice that the intensity of gesture-related PPG patterns is sensitive to the locations of sensors on the wrist, thus it may not be significant enough for segmentation. The insight is that the PPG sensors can capture more significant changes of reflected light when they are closer to the arteries that are directly compressed by muscles and tendons. Through our extensive tests, we find that two PPG sensors at a close distance on the wrist can already provide good diversity, and at least one of them can provide gesture-related PPG signals that have the stronger intensity than that of pulse-related signals. Therefore, in this work, we employ a two-sensor approach and determine which sensor could be the *Reference Sensor* having the significant gesture-related PPG patterns, which will be taken as the input for the fine-grained data segmentation. Specifically, we examine the short-time energy of the extracted PPG measurements and determine whether a sensor is a *Reference Sensor* or not depending on if its short-time energy exceeds the threshold θ.

7.6 Performance Evaluation

7.6.1 Experimental Methodology

Wearable Prototype We notice that existing manufacturers do not provide direct access to raw PPG readings; instead, they only provide computed heart rate. Therefore, we design a wearable prototype that mimics the layout of PPG sensors in commodity wearables to demonstrate that our system can be applied to the existing wearable products without extra efforts. Our prototype consists of two commodity PPG sensors (with single green LED) and an Arduino UNO (REV3) as shown in Fig. 7.9. The sensors are closely placed to each other and fixed on the inner side of a wristband, so that it reduces the movements of sensors and ensures our system to take sensor measurements at similar locations in different experiments. In the experiments, we adopt various sampling rates (i.e., 30–100 Hz) to evaluate the system. Unless mentioned otherwise, the default sampling rate is set to 100 Hz.

Data Collection We recruit 10 participants including 9 males and 1 female whose ages are between 20–30 to perform finger-level gestures for evaluation. We focus on the elementary gestures from American Sign Language involving movements of fingers from a single hand as shown in Fig. 7.10. The participants are asked to respectively perform the nine finger-level gestures for 40 times while wearing our wearable prototype on the right wrist. Note that our system can be applied to other more complicated finger-level gestures on whichever wrist regardless of the posture of the hand since different gestures involve different combinations of muscle movements that can be captured by our system. In total, we collect 3600 PPG segments for the experimental evaluation. Unless mentioned otherwise, our

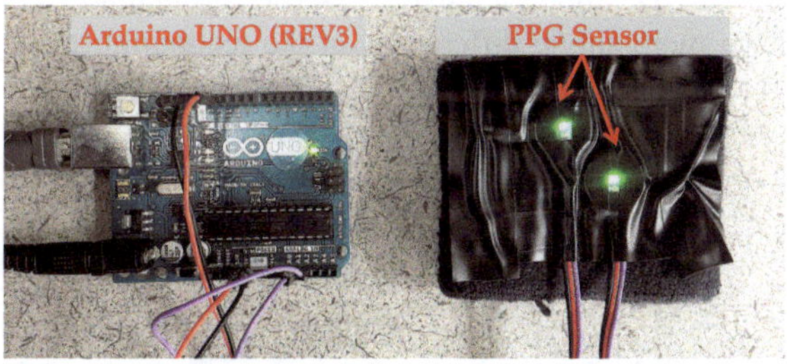

Fig. 7.9 Prototype wrist-worn PPG sensing platform

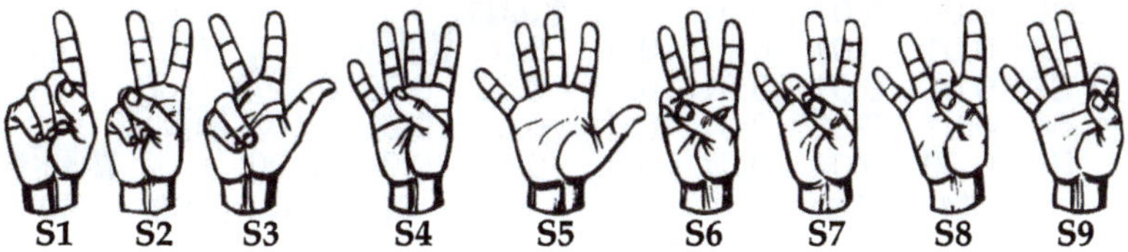

Fig. 7.10 American sign language of number one to nine

results are derived from 20 rounds Monte Carlo cross-validation using 50% of our data set for training and the rest for validation. The data are processed by our system implemented by MATLAB, which is run on an ASUS Q324U notebook.

7.6.2 Evaluation Metrics

Precision Given N_g segments of a gesture type g, precision of recognizing the gesture type g is defined as $Precision_g = N_g^T/(N_g^T + M_g^F)$, where N_g^T is the number of gesture segments correctly recognized as the gesture g. M_g^F is the number of gesture segments corresponding to other gestures which are mistakenly recognized as the gesture type g.

Recall Recall of the gesture type g is defined as the percentage of the segments that are correctly recognized as the gesture type g among all segments of the gesture type g, which is defined as $Recall_g = N_g^T/N_g$.

7.6.3 Sign Language Interpretation Performance

Figure 7.11 depicts the confusion matrix for the recognition of the nine American Sign Language gestures. Each entry C_{ij} denotes the percentage of the number of gesture segments i was predicted as gesture type j in the total number of i. The diagonal entries show the average accuracy of recognizing each gesture, respectively. Specifically, the average accuracy is 88.32% with standard deviation 2.3% among all the 9 gestures. We find that the recognition results of the gesture $S2$, $S6$, $S7$, $S8$ are relatively low (i.e., around 86%). This is because those gestures have more subtle differences in the tendon/muscle dynamics than other gestures. Overall, the results confirm that it is promising to use commodity wrist-worn PPG sensors to perform finger-level gesture recognition.

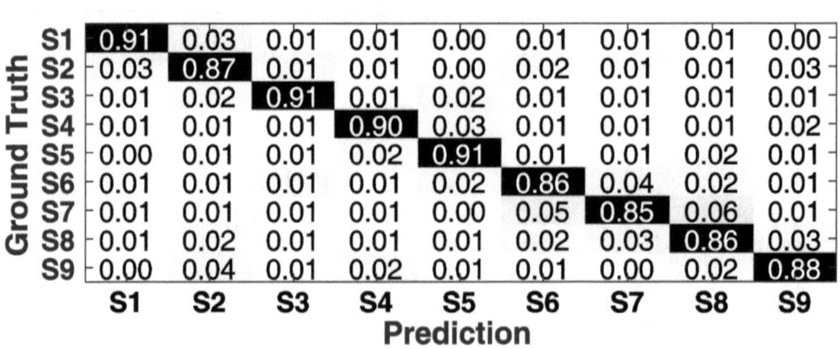

Fig. 7.11 Confusion matrix of recognizing nine finger-level gestures among ten participants

7.6.4 Study of Different Impact Factors to the System

Impact of Different Users Figure 7.12a and b present the average precision and recall of recognizing each finger-level gesture across different participants. We observe that all participants have high accuracy on recognizing these finger-level gestures. Specifically, the average precision and recall of all the 10 participants are 88% and 89%, respectively, and the lowest average value of the precision and recall among all the participants is still above 80%. The results show the robustness and scalability of our proposed system across different users, and demonstrate the system is promising to act as an integrated function in commodity wearables once the interface of PPG raw signals to developers is open.

Impact of Different Gestures We next study the impact of different sign gestures on the performance of the proposed system and show the average precision/recall for each sign gesture. As shown in Fig. 7.13a, it is encouraging to find that all those gestures can be recognized well with the lowest average precision and recall as 85 and 84%, respectively. Furthermore, Fig. 7.13b shows the standard deviation of the precision and recall of recognizing each gesture. The gestures $S1$, $S2$ and $S6$ have relatively high standard deviation. This is because participants $P2$ and $P3$ inconsistently perform $S1$, $S2$ and $S6$ respectively based on our observation. Overall, our system is robust on recognizing different finger-level gestures.

Impact of Sampling Rate The sampling rate of sensing hardware is one of the critical impact factors on affecting the power consumption of wearables, thus we study the performance of the proposed system with different sampling rates on PPG sensors. Most of the commodity wearables have around 100 Hz PPG sampling rate. For instance, Samsung Simband [22] configures its PPG sensor to 128 Hz to perform time-centric tasks (e.g., Pulse Arrival Time calculations). Therefore, we set our wearable prototype to collect PPG measurements with different sampling rates (i.e., 30–100 Hz with a step size of 20 Hz) in our experiments. Figure 7.14a shows the average precision and recall of the gesture recognition under different sampling rates. We find that the precision/recall increases with the increased sampling rate, however, the precision/recall still maintain as high as 87% at the lowest sampling rate (i.e., 30 Hz). As the results implied, our system is compatible to commodity wearables and can provide high recognition accuracy with lower PPG sampling rate in terms of the power consumption.

Impact of Training Data Size We change the percentage of data used for training in the Monte Carlo cross-validation to study the performance of our system under different training data size as shown in Fig. 7.14b. In particular, we choose the percentages 12.5, 25, 37.5, 50, and 62.5%, which correspond to 5, 10, 15, 20, and 25 PPG segments with respect to each gesture for training, and use the rest of our data for validation. We observe that our system can achieve an average precision of 75% for recognizing nine finger-level gestures using only 5 PPG segments of each gesture for training. As the size of the training data grows, the system

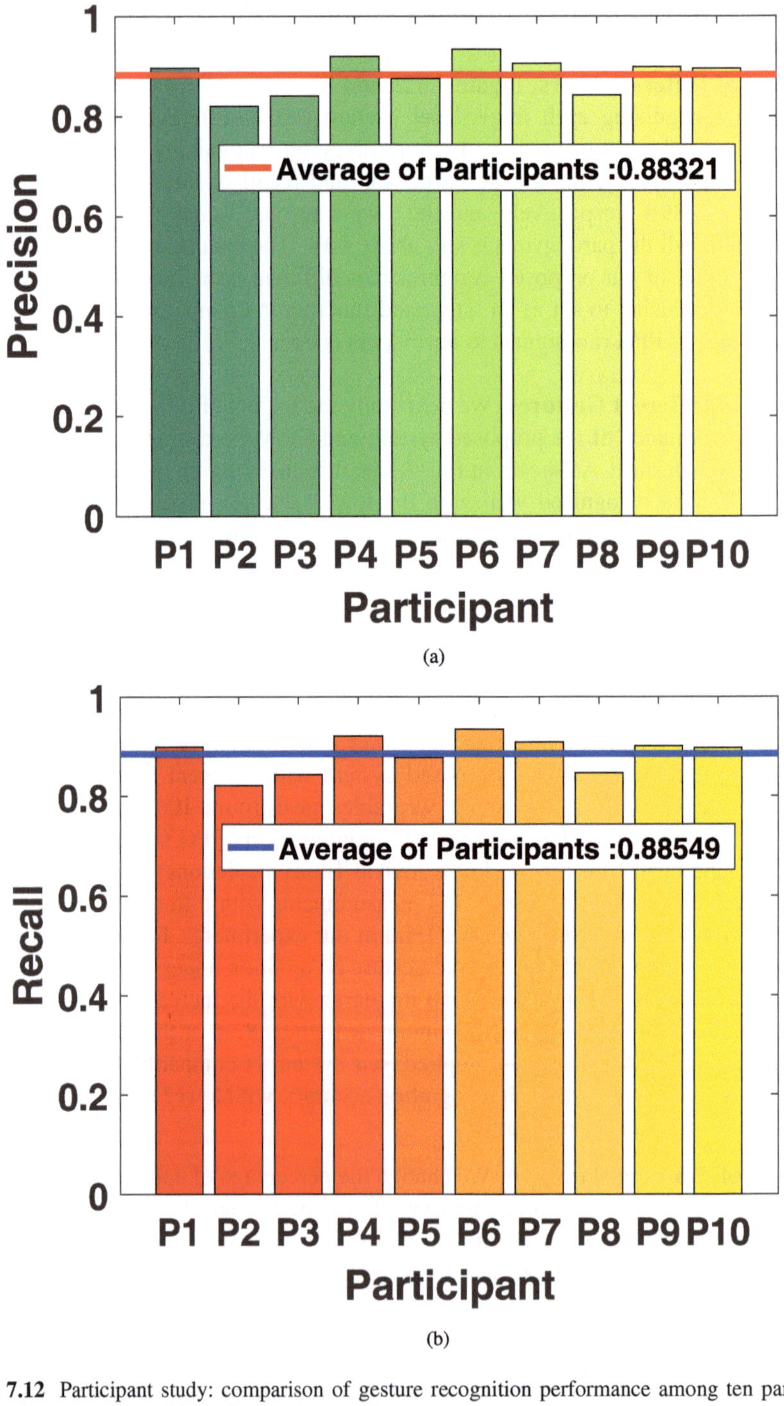

Fig. 7.12 Participant study: comparison of gesture recognition performance among ten participants. (**a**) Average precision. (**b**) Average recall

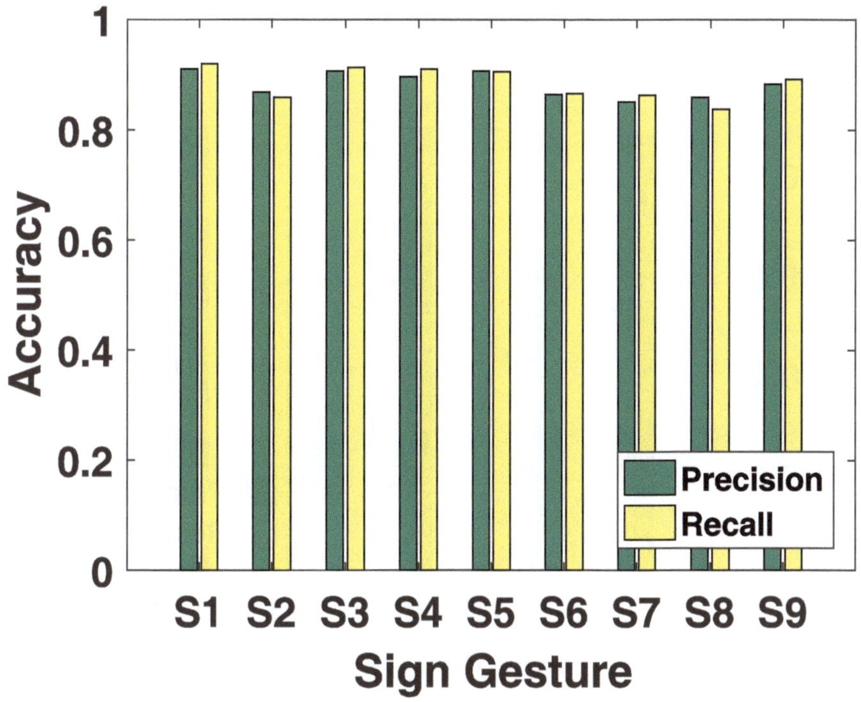

(a)

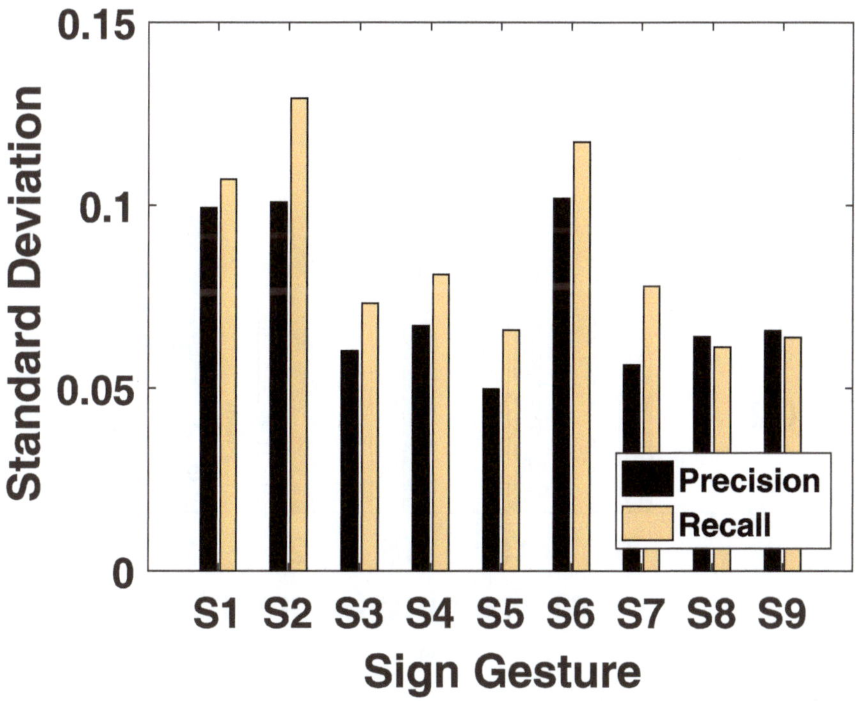

(b)

Fig. 7.13 Gesture study: Comparison of gesture recognition performance between nine gestures. (**a**) Average precision and recall. (**b**) STD of precision and recall

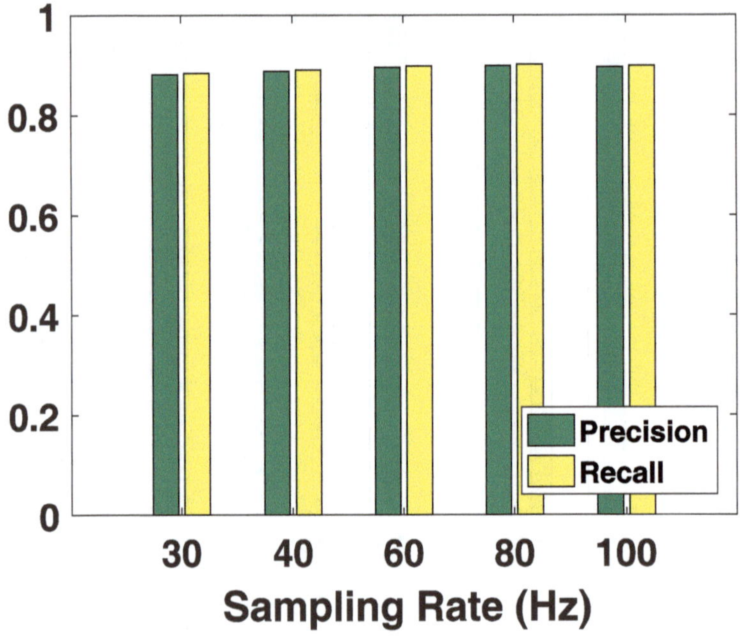

(a)

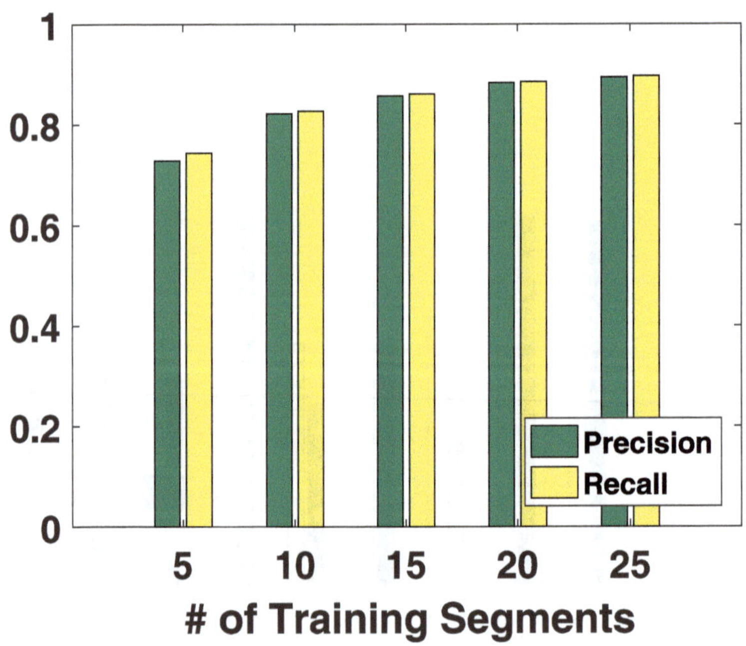

(b)

Fig. 7.14 Impact factor study: average precision and recall of recognizing nine gestures with different sampling rates and # of training segments. (**a**) Impact of sampling rate. (**b**) Impact of # of training segments

performance improves significantly. More specifically, the average precision and recall can achieve 89 and 90% respectively when 25 segments of training data for each gesture are collected in the training phase. The above results indicate our system can achieve good recognition performance with a limited size of training data (e.g., 5 sets per gesture), which ensures great convenience for practical usage on commodity wearables.

7.7 Summary

Gesture recognition, as a crucial aspect of human-computer interactions, has garnered considerable research attention in recent years. This chapter represents a significant stride towards comprehensively understanding PPG-based gesture recognition. Our work introduces an innovative approach for recognizing fine-grained finger-level gestures, including sign language, by utilizing affordable PPG sensors integrated into wearables. To achieve this, we have developed a novel proposition that effectively separates the distinctive gesture-related patterns from the continuously interfered PPG measurements, caused by pulsations. This is made possible through the implementation of a fine-grained data segmentation method. Furthermore, we have investigated the unique PPG features generated by finger-level gestures across various signal domains. Leveraging this knowledge, we have devised a system that can accurately recognize finger-level gestures solely based on PPG measurements. In our experiments, we collected and analyzed over 3600 gestures from a group of ten participants. The results demonstrate that our system achieves an impressive average recognition accuracy of over 88% when differentiating nine elementary finger-level gestures from American Sign Language. While conducting this research, we acknowledged several factors that may impact the performance of PPG sensors. For instance, we recognized that the intensity of reflected light captured by PPG sensors is sensitive to variations in skin color, with lighter skin reflecting more light. Additionally, the location of the sensor on the wrist can affect signal strength, with signals being weaker on the outer side. Moreover, strenuous physical activities can significantly influence PPG signals. These considerations necessitate further investigation and the exploration of potential solutions, such as incorporating motion sensors, to address these impact factors in our future work. By presenting our findings and actively seeking solutions for these challenges, we aim to advance the field of PPG-based gesture recognition and facilitate its practical implementation in diverse real-world scenarios.

References

1. Adib, F., Kabelac, Z., Katabi, D., Miller, R.C.: 3d tracking via body radio reflections. In: NSDI, vol. 14, pp. 317–329 (2014)

2. Adib, F., Kabelac, Z., Katabi, D.: Multi-person localization via rf body reflections. In: NSDI, pp. 279–292 (2015)
3. Ahmed, A.: Frequency of a beating heart (1998). https://hypertextbook.com/facts/1998/ArsheAhmed.shtml
4. Allen, J.: Photoplethysmography and its application in clinical physiological measurement. Physiol. Meas. **28**(3), R1 (2007)
5. Asadzadeh, P., Kulik, L., Tanin, E.: Gesture recognition using rfid technology. Pers. Ubiquitous Comput. **16**(3), 225–234 (2012)
6. Becker, C., Rigamonti, R., Lepetit, V., Fua, P.: Supervised feature learning for curvilinear structure segmentation. In: International Conference on Medical Image Computing and Computer-Assisted Intervention, pp. 526–533. Springer (2013)
7. Bombardini, T., Gemignani, V., Bianchini, E., Venneri, L., Petersen, C., Pasanisi, E., Pratali, L., Alonso-Rodriguez, D., Pianelli, M., Faita, F., et al.: Diastolic time–frequency relation in the stress echo lab: filling timing and flow at different heart rates. Cardiovasc. Ultrasound **6**(1), 15 (2008)
8. Ebrahimzadeh, E., Pooyan, M.: Early detection of sudden cardiac death by using classical linear techniques and time-frequency methods on electrocardiogram signals. J. Biomed. Sci. Eng. **4**(11), 699 (2011)
9. Friedman, J., Hastie, T., Tibshirani, R.: Regularization paths for generalized linear models via coordinate descent. J. Stat. Softw. **33**(1), 1 (2010)
10. Galar, M., Fernández, A., Barrenechea, E., Bustince, H., Herrera, F.: An overview of ensemble methods for binary classifiers in multi-class problems: Experimental study on one-vs-one and one-vs-all schemes. Pattern Recognit. **44**(8), 1761–1776 (2011)
11. Hastie, T., Tibshirani, R., Friedman, J.: The Elements of Statistical Learning, pp. 115–163. Springer, New York (2001)
12. Innerbody.com: Flexor digitorum superficialis muscle (2017). http://www.innerbody.com/image_musc05/musc50.html
13. Klostermann, J.: Blinging up fashionable wearable technologies (2015). https://cloudtweaks.com/2015/11/blinging-up-fashionable-wearable-technologies/
14. Li, T., An, C., Tian, Z., Campbell, A.T., Zhou, X.: Human sensing using visible light communication. In: Proceedings of the 21st Annual International Conference on Mobile Computing and Networking, pp. 331–344. ACM (2015)
15. Lu, Z., Chen, X., Li, Q., Zhang, X., Zhou, P.: A hand gesture recognition framework and wearable gesture-based interaction prototype for mobile devices. IEEE Trans. Human-Mach. Syst. **44**(2), 293–299 (2014)
16. Mao, W., He, J., Qiu, L.: Cat: high-precision acoustic motion tracking. In: Proceedings of the 22nd Annual International Conference on Mobile Computing and Networking, pp. 69–81. ACM (2016)
17. Marin, G., Dominio, F., Zanuttigh, P.: Hand gesture recognition with leap motion and kinect devices. In: 2014 IEEE International Conference on Image Processing (ICIP), pp. 1565–1569. IEEE (2014)
18. Nandakumar, R., Iyer, V., Tan, D., Gollakota, S.: Fingerio: Using active sonar for fine-grained finger tracking. In: Proceedings of the 2016 CHI Conference on Human Factors in Computing Systems, pp. 1515–1525. ACM (2016)
19. Noei, S., Ashtari, P., Jahed, M., Vahdat, B.V.: Classification of eeg signals using the spatio-temporal feature selection via the elastic net. In: 2016 23rd Iranian Conference on Biomedical Engineering and 2016 1st International Iranian Conference on Biomedical Engineering (ICBME), pp. 232–236. IEEE (2016)
20. Pu, Q., Gupta, S., Gollakota, S., Patel, S.: Whole-home gesture recognition using wireless signals. In: Proceedings of the 19th Annual International Conference on Mobile Computing & Networking, pp. 27–38. ACM (2013)
21. Ren, Z., Yuan, J., Meng, J., Zhang, Z.: Robust part-based hand gesture recognition using kinect sensor. IEEE Trans. Multimedia **15**(5), 1110–1120 (2013)

22. Simband: Why is 128 hz used as a sampling frequency for the ppg signals? (2017). http://www.simband.io/documentation/faq.html
23. Sun, L., Sen, S., Koutsonikolas, D., Kim, K.H.: Widraw: enabling hands-free drawing in the air on commodity wifi devices. In: Proceedings of the 21st Annual International Conference on Mobile Computing and Networking, pp. 77–89. ACM (2015)
24. Sznitman, R., Becker, C., Fleuret, F., Fua, P.: Fast object detection with entropy-driven evaluation. In: Proceedings of the IEEE Conference on Computer Vision and Pattern Recognition, pp. 3270–3277 (2013)
25. Tamura, T., Maeda, Y., Sekine, M., Yoshida, M.: Wearable photoplethysmographic sensors-past and present. Electronics **3**(2), 282–302 (2014)
26. Vuksanovic, B., Alhamdi, M.: Ar-based method for ecg classification and patient recognition. Int. J. Biom. Bioinform. **7**(2), 74 (2013)
27. Wang, H., Lai, T.T.T., Roy Choudhury, R.: Mole: Motion leaks through smartwatch sensors. In: Proceedings of the 21st Annual International Conference on Mobile Computing and Networking, pp. 155–166. ACM (2015)
28. Xu, C., Pathak, P.H., Mohapatra, P.: Finger-writing with smartwatch: a case for finger and hand gesture recognition using smartwatch. In: Proceedings of the 16th International Workshop on Mobile Computing Systems and Applications, pp. 9–14. ACM (2015)
29. Zhang, X., Chen, X., Li, Y., Lantz, V., Wang, K., Yang, J.: A framework for hand gesture recognition based on accelerometer and emg sensors. IEEE Trans. Syst. Man Cybern. Part A Syst. Humans **41**(6), 1064–1076 (2011)
30. Zhang, Y., Harrison, C.: Tomo: wearable, low-cost electrical impedance tomography for hand gesture recognition. In: Proceedings of the 28th Annual ACM Symposium on User Interface Software & Technology, pp. 167–173. ACM (2015)

Chapter 8
Continuous User Authentication via PPG

PPG technology offers potentials not only in sign language interpretation, but also in user authentication. Traditional single-instance user authentication methods often result in a less-than-ideal user experience, especially in frequently used applications. This problem is notably acute in security-sensitive contexts, where unauthorized access could potentially follow a user's initial login. In response to this, continuous user authentication (CA) has emerged as a compelling solution, offering seamless, low-effort authentication for users. In this chapter, we present a cost-effective system that leverages pulsatile signals captured by the photoplethysmography (PPG) sensor in commercially available wrist-worn wearables for CA. Our system stands out by eliminating the need for users' participations and accommodating non-clinical PPG measurements that are prone to motion artifacts (MA), commonly encountered during daily activities. To address the challenges posed by MA, we delve into the unique characteristics of the human cardiac system and propose an MA filtering method that effectively mitigates the impact of everyday movements. Moreover, we identify key fiducial features and develop an adaptive classifier using the gradient boosting tree (GBT) method. Consequently, our system can continuously authenticate users based on their cardiac characteristics, requiring minimal training effort. We conduct experiments with our wrist-worn PPG sensing platform in practical scenarios. The results demonstrate the high accuracy of our system and a low false detection rate when detecting random attacks. The structure of the remainder of this chapter is as follows. Section 8.1 introduces the research background to provide the context for this study. Section 8.2, reviews the current literature related to the field of continuous user authentication via PPG on smartwatches. In Sect. 8.3, we delve into the feasibility of such authentication system, describing the attack model, system design, PPG feature extraction and authentication, and general wrist PPG feature extraction. Section 8.4 deals with the challenge of motion artifacts, exploring their detection, classification, removal for near-wrist activities and mitigation for far-wrist activities. In Sect. 8.5, we provide

X. Guo et al., *Mobile Technologies for Smart Healthcare System Design*,
Wireless Networks, https://doi.org/10.1007/978-3-031-57345-3_8

a thorough depiction of the system's implementation, including data preprocessing and pulse segmentation. Section 8.6 encompasses the system's performance evaluation, covering experimental methodology, evaluation metrics, continuous authentication performance, impact of various factors, CA performance with motion artifacts removal and mitigation, and effectiveness of adaptive training. Finally, Sect. 8.7 concludes the chapter with a succinct summary.

8.1 Background

Traditional user authentication methods rely on users' inputs, such as passwords and graphic patterns. However, these methods are known to be vulnerable to many attacks [2, 19]. Recently, multi-factor authentication (MFA) [4, 24] has been proposed to mitigate these threats by verifying two or more types of confidential information from independent sources. While many applications have adopted either one-factor or MFA, both of these two approaches use a one-time login process, which is not secure enough to authenticate users during certain applications. This is especially critical for a security-sensitive application, in which an adversary could obtain unauthorized privileges after a user's initial login. Therefore, a practical continuous user authentication (CA) solution that can periodically verify a user's identity without interruptions of the application usage is highly in demand [1].

Existing CA approaches usually focus on reducing or eliminating user involvement in the authentication process by leveraging users' unique behavioral patterns. For example, keystroke/mouse dynamics [21, 33] and gait patterns [29] have been used for user authentication since 2012. These approaches usually rely on momentary events and can only determine a user's identity by monitoring particular activities (e.g., typing, mouse-clicking, or walking). There are studies using cardiac signals (e.g., ECG [14, 26] and cardiac motion [20]) for CA. All these systems require dedicated sensors (e.g., ECG or Doppler radar sensors), which are costly and not readily available in commodity devices. Recently, researchers find that the photoplethysmography (PPG) sensor can also provide unique cardiac biometric information for user authentication [6, 15, 16, 30]. However, these systems only focus on clinical scenarios, under which strong and stable PPG measurements are collected from the fingertips of static subjects.

Different from the existing works, we develop a low-cost CA system, which can periodically verify the identity of a user via cardiac signals (i.e., PPG) from common wrist-worn wearable devices (e.g., smartwatches and fitness trackers). Under a working environment shown in Fig. 8.1a, our system can continuously determine whether a current staff operating a specific device (e.g., a smartphone or a laptop) is a legitimate user in a non-intrusive manner so that any time-sensitive tasks will not be interrupted. As a result, a user can continuously trade stocks, manage air traffic, or switch circuits. As a daily life example in Fig. 8.1b, each family member with a wearable device can be periodically authenticated by the system so that he/she can enjoy a seamless experience of accessing or switching between user-specific

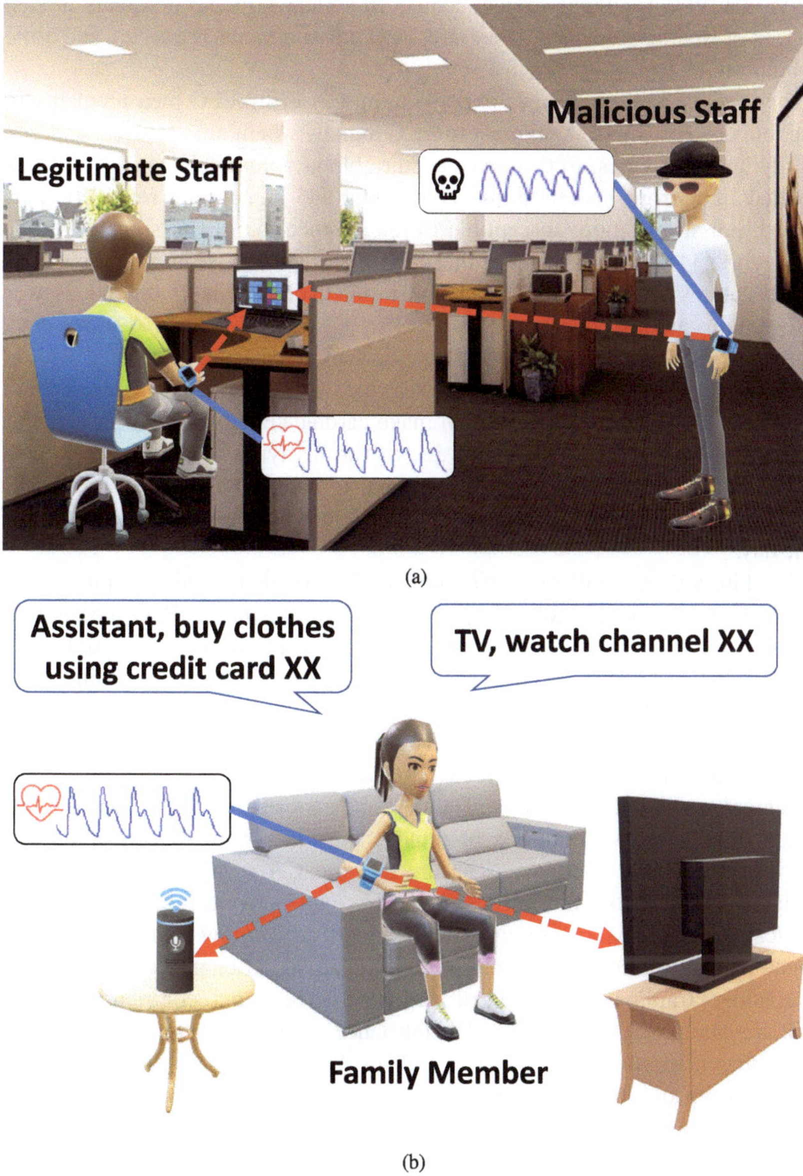

Fig. 8.1 Two scenarios of continuous user authentication (CA). (**a**) CA in office scenarios. (**b**) CA in living scenarios

apps on the smart devices paired with the system. Therefore, each person can watch his/her own favorite channels in a smart TV or do online shopping via a voice assistant. The advantage of using PPG for CA is obvious as cardiac signals are unique and ever-present biometrics which are available without users' involvement.

In addition, PPG requires physical contact to human skin and is usually hidden in the back of wearable devices. Therefore, PPG measurements are secure and difficult to counterfeit.

There are several challenges in performing CA using PPG measurements from wearable devices. First, in contrast to ECG signals which are electrical and generated by heart activities, PPG signals capture blood volume changes by measuring reflected light from human skins. Therefore, PPG signals are relatively coarse-grained, noisy, and more susceptible to interference than ECG signals. Although initial works [18, 30] have shown that PPG measurements from fingertips contain unique features to be used for user authentication in clinical environments. However, these features are not persistent in the PPG signals collected from wearable devices in practice. Second, wrist-worn wearable devices are usually associated with a lot of hand or body movements from daily activities. These movements would result in various motion artifacts (MAs) which make cardiac signals in PPG measurements often unavailable in practice. Third, due to various types of imprecisions in PPG sensors in wearable devices and loose contacts between them and human skins, cardiac signals from PPG measurements could vary in different days or even in the same day.

To address these challenges, we particularly investigate and determine *general fiducial features* that are not only persistent in various users' PPG measurements but also can capture unique characteristics of cardiac motions for CA. Additionally, we study the MAs of different types of body-movements (e.g., walking, moving forearm, and drinking water) in practical scenarios and categorize them into two types: *far-wrist* and *near-wrist*, based on the recoverability of cardiac signals with the MAs. We further develop effective *MA detection* and *MA mitigation/removal mechanisms* to identify the two type of MAs and choose to either recover the cardiac signals from weak MA impacts or remove the measurements containing strong MA impacts. These mechanisms ensure that our CA system can extract correct cardiac signals without the impact from MAs and perform CA accurately under practical scenarios. Moreover, our system adopts an *adaptive updating mechanism* to automatically accommodate the user's cardiac signal changes over time based on adaptive training of associated classifiers. The main contributions of this work are summarized as follows. We introduce a pioneering low-cost continuous user authentication (CA) system that utilizes unique cardiac biometrics extracted from PPG sensors in wrist-worn wearable devices, specifically designed for easy integration with PPG-enabled wearables like smartwatches. Our research involves an extensive exploration of motion artifacts (MAs) in real-world scenarios, leading to the development of robust mechanisms for MA mitigation and removal. These mechanisms effectively identify various types and intensities of MAs, ensuring minimal impact on authentication accuracy. Through the identification of general fiducial features, we capture the individuality of users' cardiac patterns, enabling the creation of an adaptive gradient boosting tree (GBT)-based classifier that remains resilient to signal drifts in PPG, thereby ensuring reliable user authentication and effective defense against random attacks. To validate our approach, we implement a prototype of the proposed system using commercially available PPG sensors and conduct experiments involving 20 participants. The results demonstrate our system's exceptional performance, with an average CA accuracy surpassing 90% and a low false detection rate of 4% when detecting random attacks.

8.2 Related Work

Recent user authentication systems often use users' biometrics (e.g., behavioral or physiological information) to reduce user involvement and facilitate CA. Behavioral pattern is considered a distinct biometric that can make CA possible based on users' daily activities. For example, Mondol et al. [22] propose a user authentication system leveraging motion sensors in smartwatches to capture users' signatures in the air for authentication. Casale et al. [8] develop a wearable-based authentication system based on users' walk patterns. However, these approaches rely on users' involvement in specific activities in such a great deal to easily cause inconvenience.

Physiological-based biometrics (e.g., cardiac and respiratory motions) are popularly used for building CA systems because they can be obtained without users' active participation. For instance, Lin et al. [20] propose a CA system, Cardiac Scan, which utilizes DC-coupled continuous-wave radar to capture distinct heart motions in the user identification process. Rahman et al. [28] develop a method that uses the Doppler radar to identify users based on their respiratory motions. Although these systems provide a sound foundation for CA using wireless technology, they use dedicated devices that might not be available for users yet. Recently advanced sensing technologies enable unobtrusive and continuous user authentication based on unique cardiac biometrics captured by electrocardiogram (ECG) sensors [7, 12]. While mostly available under clinical environments, these systems require users to wear electrodes at various locations. This again turns out to be inconvenient for the uses in practice.

Unlike ECG, PPG is widely used in commodity wearable devices such as smartwatches and fitness trackers. Some initial studies have explored PPG-based authentications. For example, fiducial features [6, 30] have been discovered to capture unique characteristics in human cardiac systems so they can facilitate user authentication processes. Recently, non-fiducial features (i.e., discrete wavelet transform (DWT) coefficients) of PPG signals are proposed to build CA systems [15, 16]. However, all of the aforementioned studies collect PPG measurements from users' fingertips thus require users to wear dedicated PPG sensors and keep motionless. These requirements are difficult to meet in reality.

Different from the existing work, we build the first low-cost PPG-based system that can perform CA in practical scenarios with various body movements by leveraging PPG sensors in commodity wrist-worn devices. We identify general fiducial features that can capture distinct cardiac biometrics of diverse PPG measurements collected from users' wrist areas. In addition, we extensively study the impact of motions with different intensities and develop the MA removal method that can effectively remove MA and significantly improve the CA performance. Moreover, our system employs an adaptive user authentication method that can reduce the impact of system drifts and provide long-term PPG-based CA.

8.3 Continuous User Authentication via PPG on Smartwatches

8.3.1 Attack Model

We assume that attackers cannot compromise users' wearable devices (i.e., gaining access to their memory storages for raw PPG measurements). Based on this, the possible attacks to our CA system are as follows:

Random Attack Attackers or their accomplices wear users' wearable devices and expect the PPG measurements captured can pass our PPG-based CA system. This random attack model is similar to the brute-force attack.

Synthesis Attack To launch this attack, attackers first need to obtain users' blood flow patterns through either medical records or vision-based technologies (e.g., remote photoplethysmography (rPPG) [23]). However, these patterns and the PPG measurements collected from users' wrist areas are different in collection approaches and conditions. In addition, the PPG signals are collected in an enclosed environment (between the back of wearable devices and skin contact areas) so that many critical measurement data (light absorption/reflection of human skin, light source intensity, etc.) As a result, synthesis attacks will not be easily launched.

8.3.2 Feasibility Study of Using PPG for User Authentication

Intuition of Using Wearable PPG for CA Human cardiac systems have been studied and known to be distinct among people [31]. Along this direction, initial studies [18, 30] have shown that *fiducial features* derived from critical landmarks in the raw PPG measurements and their derivatives (i.e., the systolic/diastolic peaks, dicrotic notch, and points a/b/c in Fig. 8.2) can be used as users' unique biometric information. However, these studies only analyze PPG data collected from clinical settings with quite strict requirements. Thus, how to design and realize a PPG-based CA system using wrist-worn devices in practices remains a challenging task.

Difference Between Wrist-Worn PPG and Fingertip PPG To illustrate such a difference, we collect PPG measurements from both fingertip and wrist areas of the same users simultaneously using our prototype PPG sensing platform. The top two panels of Fig. 8.3 show that the PPG measurements from the wrist area are stable but

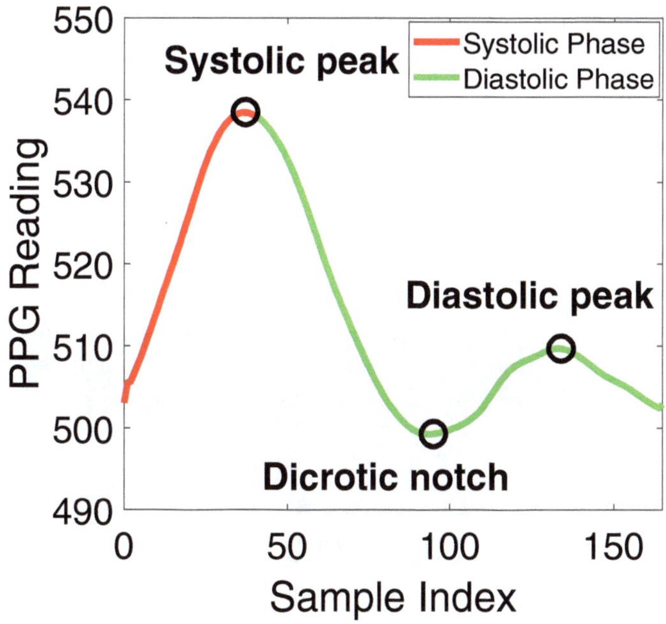

(a)

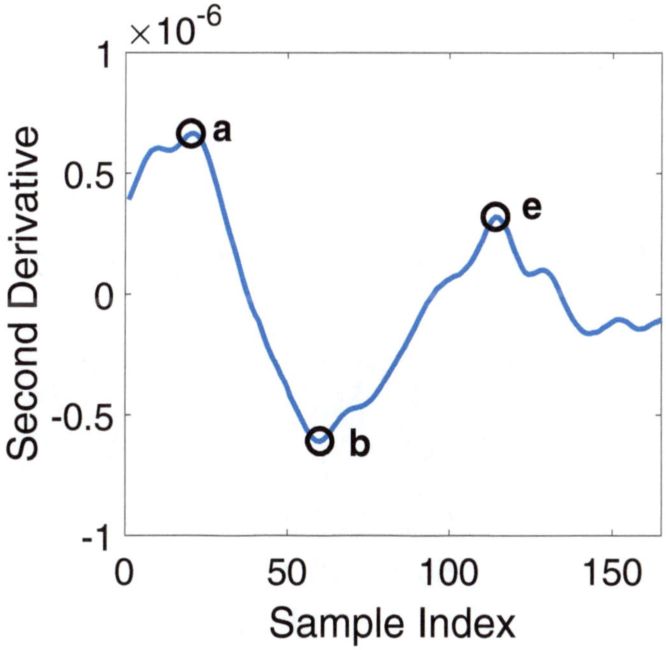

(b)

Fig. 8.2 Illustration of the critical landmarks in raw PPG measurements and its second derivative. (**a**) Raw PPG measurements. (**b**) Second derivative of raw PPG measurements

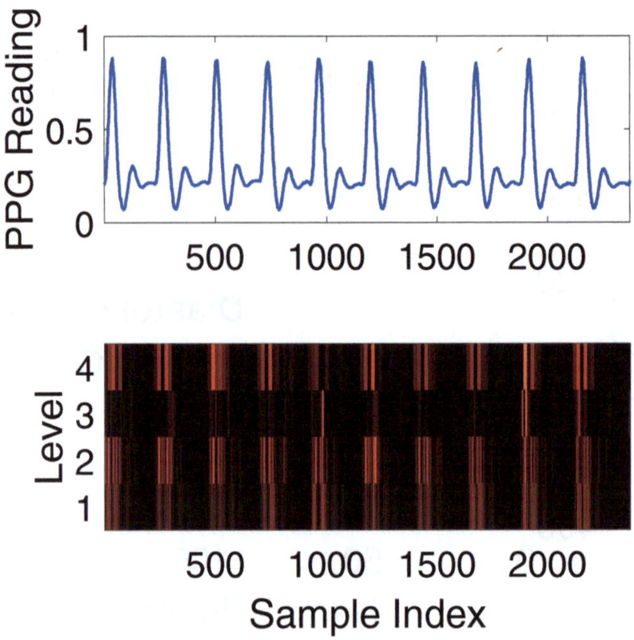

(a)

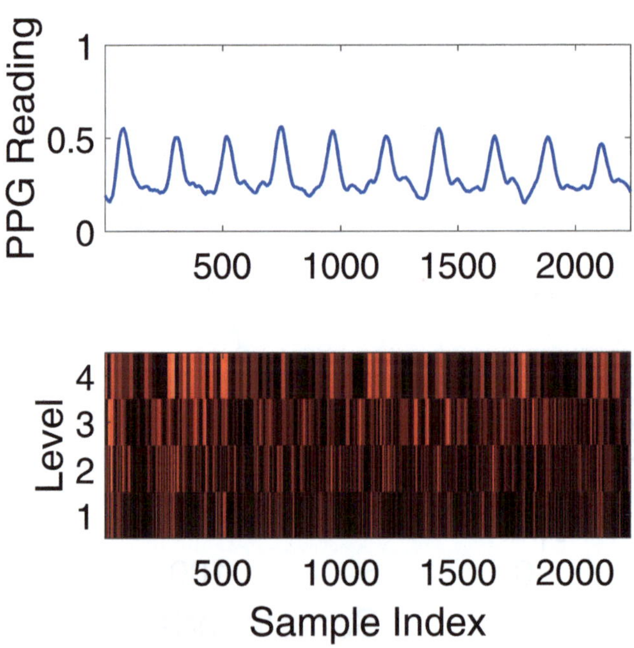

(b)

Fig. 8.3 Example of PPG data from fingertip and wrist and their corresponding discrete wavelet transform. (**a**) Fingertip PPG data and DWT coefficients. (**b**) Wrist PPG data and DWT coefficients

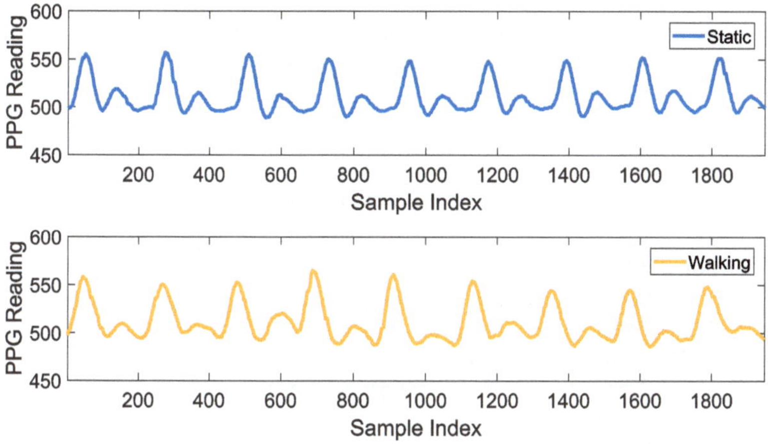

Fig. 8.4 The PPG measurements of the same people under static scenario and walking scenario

with less detectable and critical landmarks than those from the fingertip area. This indicates that the existing fiducial-feature-based authentication approaches [18, 30] are not applicable directly to the PPG from wearable devices. We further generate non-fiducial feature for both PPG measurements using the Daubechies wavelet of order 4 (db4) with four levels of decomposition. The bottom two panels in Fig. 8.3 show that the fingertip PPG readings have repetitive and stable DWT coefficients with respect to each heartbeat in four levels, whereas the wrist area PPG readings are embedded with many noisy and irregular DWT coefficients, which will significantly impact the performance of the non-fiducial-based PPG authentication work [15, 16]. Therefore, instead of adopting non-fiducial features, there is a need to explore more general fiducial features in the PPG signal from the wrist area for CA.

Impact of Daily Activities To better understand the impact of daily activities as motion artifacts (MAs), we categorize them into three types based on the different moving parts of human bodies involved: *far-wrist*, *near-wrist*, and *whole-body* activities. The far-wrist activities are the major arm movements without involving tendons and muscles of the wrist area. In contrast, the near-wrist activities are finger-level and/or wrist-level movements, which have direct impacts on blood volume changes in the wrist area and more significant impact on PPG measurements from wearable devices. The whole-body activities are associated with most of human body parts. We find that some whole-body activities of low intensity, such as leisure walking, do not have noticeable impacts on the PPG measurements as shown in Fig. 8.4. More strenuous activities, such as running, would change PPG readings significantly. In this work, we focus on the static and moving scenarios involving far-wrist and near-wrist activities, which cover the main scenarios in CA. We present the detailed design of our system in the following sections.

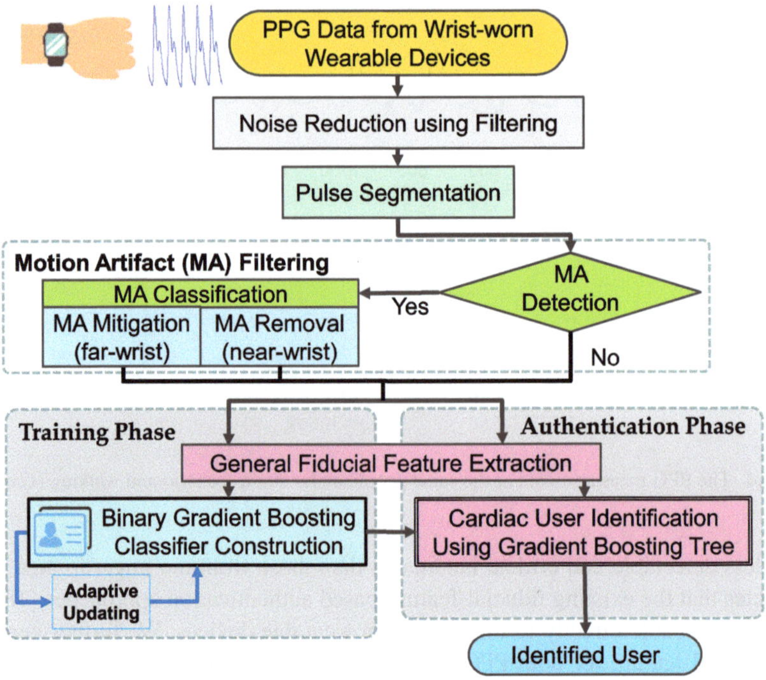

Fig. 8.5 Architecture of of the proposed user authentication using PPG

8.3.3 PPG-based Authentication System Design

The architecture of our PPG-based continuous user authentication system is shown in Fig. 8.5. The system collects PPG measurements constantly from users' wearable devices as the input. Due to hardware imperfection, the raw PPG measurements inevitably contain baseline drifts and high-frequency interferences. Therefore, our system first performs *Noise Reduction using Filtering* to reduce such impacts. A band-pass filter is used to extract pulsatile components in PPG measurements. After filtering, the system conducts *Pulse Segmentation* to determine the PPG segment that is likely to contain a complete cardiac cycle. The insight is that each cardiac cycle should include a *systolic peak*, which could be identified in the PPG measurement during typical diastole and systole phases.

Next, we design *Motion Artifact (MA) Filtering* to remove MAs caused by daily physical activities. In PPG measurements, MAs arise from tissue deformations and local blood flow changes in the wrist area. While pulsatile signals are repetitive in PPG measurements, most MAs have burst PPG waveforms. We calculate statistical measures, such as kurtosis, skewness, and standard deviation, in pulse waveforms and MA signals to determine whether a PPG segment contains a pulse or an MA in the *MA detection* process. If MAs are detected, our system performs *MA*

Classification to further decide whether they are from far-wrist activities or near-wrist activities. In general, near-wrist activities result in long-duration and strong and unrecoverable effects on PPG measurements, while far-wrist activities have small and recoverable impacts. When MAs are detected in many consecutive PPG segments, our system attributes them to near-wrist activities and then perform *MA Removal* to eliminate the impacted PPG segments. On the contrary, if MAs are detected in scattered or only a few consecutive segments, our system associates them with far-wrist activities and performs *MA Mitigation* to reconstruct related pulse waveforms. After the *Motion Artifact (MA) Filtering*, the data processing of our system is separated into two phases: *Training Phase* and *Authentication Phase*.

Training Phase In this phase, our system performs *General Fiducial Feature Extraction* to extract the unique cardiac features from the PPG segment and its second derivative. This process applies to both wrist PPG measurements and fingertip ones. Next, we perform *Binary Gradient Boosting Classifier Construction* to train a binary classifier for each user. In particular, we construct a user's profile based on some extracted features and use the Gradient Boosting Tree (GBT) in training the classifier when the user enrolls in the system. Furthermore, our system regularly updates the classifier with new training data to accommodate PPG drifts over time in *Adaptive Updating*.

Authentication Phase In the *Authentication Phase*, our system collects PPG segments in real-time and determines whether a current user is legitimate based on the PPG segments in a sliding window. Specifically, after our system filters MAs out from the PPG segments, it would further extract general fiducial features. Then our system performs *Cardiac User Identification Using Gradient Boosting Tree* by using the binary gradient boosting classifiers generated in the training phase to determine the user's identity based on each PPG segment. Finally, our system utilizes a majority-vote rule on the classified results of the PPG segments in the sliding-window to perform CA. In addition, our CA system is suitable for commodity wearable devices since their PPG sensors consume low power (e.g. 4mA) compared to battery capacities of these devices.

Accurate Sensing Using Low-cost PPG Sensor on the Wrist The low-cost PPG sensors in commodity wearable devices collect data from users' wrists at lower sampling rates with more noise and lower resolution. This will reduce the accuracy in user authentication.

Robust CA with Body Movements in Daily Activities The PPG sensors in the wrist-worn wearable device are particularly susceptible to daily physical activities. Therefore we need to explore characteristics of MAs from the PPG measurement and develop technologies to effectively reduce such impacts.

Effective Feature Set for General PPG Measurements The PPG measurements from the wrist area are unstable and weak, leading to fewer detectable fiducial features. Thus, we need to exam general effective features for CA.

Persistent User Authentication Against PPG Drifts The typical system-drifts in PPG sensors which could significantly impact the CA performance. Our system should study these drifts and adaptively accommodate the resulting PPG variations during a long time period.

8.3.4 PPG Feature Extraction and User Authentication

In this section, we explore the cardiac features extracted from PPG measurements and present the details of our adaptive user authentication using gradient boosting.

8.3.4.1 General Wrist PPG Feature Extraction

We have shown that the PPG measurements from the wrist area have fewer fiducial features and non-fiducial features compared to the PPG measurements from the fingertip. Therefore, we explore the fiducial features that are still available in the PPG measurements from the wrist area based on the 29 fiducial features that have been used for user authentication [10, 18].

General Wrist PPG Fiducial Features Based on our experiments with 20 participants, we find that 60% of the PPG measurements from the wrist area have only one obvious systolic peak in a cardiac cycle. To let our CA system generally work for various types of PPG measurements, we select to use five fiducial features that only require a single systolic peak in the PPG measurements. Figure 8.6 illustrates how to derive the five fiducial features from the critical landmarks in the PPG pulse waveform. The five fiducial features are generally effective for the user authentication because they are always available regardless of the source of the PPG measurements (i.e., from the wrist area or the fingertip), and they have the physiological relationships with human cardiac systems. We summarize the five fiducial features and their physiological meanings as shown in Table 8.1. Note that the five general fiducial features are always available in the PPG measurements from the fingertip. Therefore, our CA system is also applicable to the clinical PPG measurements.

8.3.4.2 Adaptive Cardiac Authentication Using Gradient Boosting Tree

Next, we build the binary classifier using Gradient Boost Tree (GBT) for user authentication. Comparing to other machine learning methods, GBT can handle the mixed types of the features with different scales, which is exactly what our general fiducial feature set possesses. Moreover, GBT is robust against the outliers via the robust loss functions and can eliminate the requirement of normalizing or whitening the feature data before classification [13].

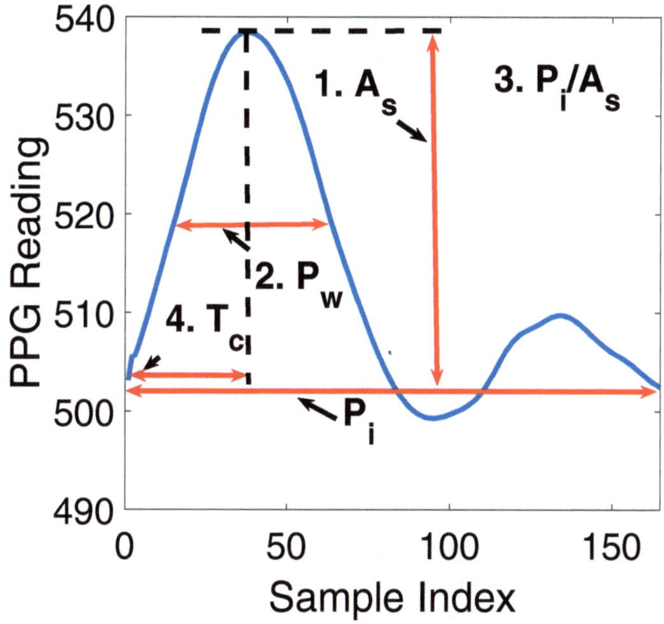

(a)

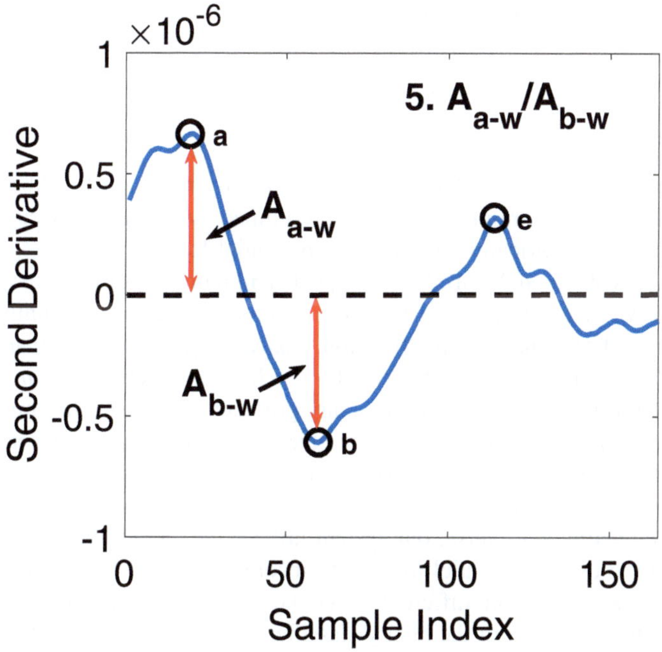

(b)

Fig. 8.6 Comparison of the Short Time Energy (STE) of the Magnitude of Linear Acceleration (MLA) and the exercise form scores on the workout review plane of user A. (**a**) Raw PPG measurements. (**b**) Second derivative of raw PPG measurements

Table 8.1 List of general wrist PPG features

Feature name	Feature description
Systolic amplitude (A_s)	Related to the stroke volume and directly proportional to vascular distensibility, which is distinguishable among different people.
Pulse width (P_w)	The width of the PPG signal at the half-height of the systolic peak, and it correlates with the systemic vascular resistance.
Ratio of pulse interval to systolic amplitude (P_i/A_s)	Reflects the functionality of a person's cardiovascular system.
Crest time (T_c)	Indicates the pulse wave velocity, which is distinct from person to person.
Ratio of amplitude of b-wave and a-wave (A_{b-w}/A_{a-w})	Reflects the arterial stiffness and the distensibility of the peripheral artery, which are also different among people. In addition, this feature can also reflect the healthy level of different people.

Specifically, given N training samples $(x_i, y_i), i = 1, \ldots, N$, where x_i and y_i represent the cardiac-related feature set and the corresponding identity label of the user (i.e., $y_i = 1$ or -1 represents whether x_i is from the current legitimate user), GBT seeks a function $\phi(x_i) = \sum_{m=1}^{M} \omega_m h_m(x_i)$ to iteratively select weak learners $h_m(\cdot)$ and their weights ω_j to minimize a loss function as follows:

$$\mathbf{L} = \sum_{i=1}^{N} L(y_i, \phi x_i). \tag{8.1}$$

We specifically adopt the GBT implementation from the SQBlib library [3] for cardiac-related feature training. In order to optimize the speed and accuracy of the GBT model, we empirically choose the exponential loss $L = e^{y_i \phi(x_i)}$ as the loss function $L(\cdot)$ with enough shrinkage (i.e., 0.1) and number of iterations (i.e., $M =$ 2000), and we take a fraction of 0.5 as the sub-sampling of the training dataset. Once we have determined the loss function, next we will construct a binary gradient classifier $b_k(\cdots)$ for each user $g_k, k = 1, \cdots, K$ to complete the *Training Phase*. Then for the testing feature set, each binary gradient classifier will output a score. The reason to use binary classifier is that binary classifier has higher accuracy in differentiating one user from other users [11] which exactly meets the fundamental requirement of a CA system.

In the *authentication phase*, our system utilizes the already-built binary classifiers for all the users in parallel to classify incoming cardiac-related feature set x. In particular, we will obtain different confidence scores from each binary classifier, and choose the identity k of the binary classifier $b_k(x)$ with the highest score as the final classification. After the user classification, we adopt a non-overlapped sliding window-based approach to perform CA. In particular, we consider P continuous PPG segments in a sliding window as a basic CA unit and use the majority vote from the classification results of these PPG segments to determine the user's identity periodically. If a half or more of the PPG segments in the window are classified to be the same user, the system would allow the current user to pass the user authentication. Otherwise, the current user does not pass the user authentication. Unless mentioned elsewhere, we use the set the sliding window size to 4 PPG segments, which generally provides good performance as shown in our evaluation.

Adaptive Updating We find that people's pulse patterns may slightly vary during a day. Therefore, we design our system to re-train the underlying classifier based on recently collected PPG measurements after each successful user authentication. Specifically, our system regularly adds a small amount of the user's PPG measurements (e.g., 2 min) to the training data to re-train a new classifier for the user in the background. This re-training process will stop until the new classifier meets the performance requirement (e.g., when the CA accuracy reaches 90%), and the new classifier will take effect until the next time re-training process starts.

8.4 Motion Artifacts Detection and Filtering to Improve System Performance

In this section, we present the MA detection and classification methods. Based on different causes of MA, we present the details of the MA removal and MA mitigation.

8.4.1 Motion Artifacts Detection

After the pulse segmentation, the system first needs to detect whether MA is affecting the PPG segments or not. We find that when there is no MA, the PPG segments should contain similar pulse waveform, thus the statistics of each PPG segment should be stable over time. However, when the PPG segments are affected by MA, the statistics of PPG measurements vary a lot. Therefore, we propose to examine the statistics of each PPG segment and use a threshold-based approach to detect the existence of MA.

In particular, we choose three types of statistics (i.e., kurtosis, skewness, and standard deviation (STD)) efficiently measuring the symmetry, tails, and dispersion of the PPG segments respectively, which are used to effectively detect MA in existing work [27]. For each type of statistics, we derive its cumulative distribution function (CDF) based on high-quality PPG segments (about 20 s) without MA. From the CDF, we determine two thresholds that can include 95% of the values of particular statistics. The statistics of the testing PPG segments will be compared to the thresholds, respectively. If any of the three types of statistics from a PPG segment is out of the range determined by the corresponding two thresholds, the PPG segment is determined to be affected by MA. Figure 8.7 presents an example

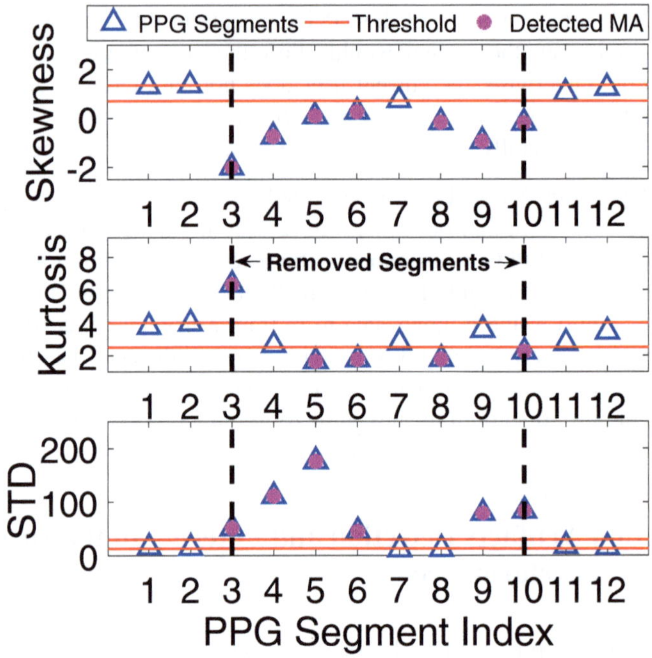

(a)

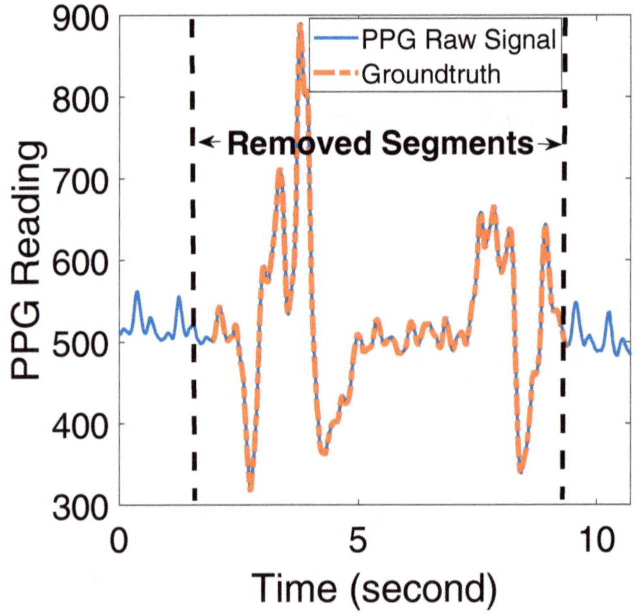

(b)

Fig. 8.7 Performance of MA detection and MA removal for the near-wrist activity. (**a**) MA detection in a sliding window for the near-wrist activity. (**b**) The PPG measurements after MA detection and removal for the near-wrist activity

of our MA detection, which shows that our method can successfully detect the PPG segments affected by MA through the three types of statistics of the PPG segments in a sliding window. We note that the accuracy of our MA detection method is over 95% in our data from the wrist collected in the moving-scenario.

8.4.2 Motion Artifacts Classification

The far-wrist activities (e.g., moving the forearm to reach a cup) usually create sparse and mild MA to PPG measurements, while the near-wrist activities (e.g., grabbing a cup) result in much stronger MA for a considerably longer period. Based on this observation, we develop an MA classification method, which examines the proportion of the PPG segments affected by MA in the sliding window $\mathcal{W}$ and determines whether the cause of MA is the near-wrist activities or far-wrist activities using a threshold-based approach. More specific, we denote the number of PPG segments that are determined to be affected and not affected by MA in the sliding window as M_W and N_W, respectively. The proportion of the PPG segments affected by MA in the sliding window is defined as the ratio $\lambda = \frac{M_W}{N_W}$. Next, λ is compared to a threshold θ_{ma}. The cause of MA is classified as the near-wrist activities if λ is greater or equal to θ_{ma}. Otherwise, the cause of MA is classified as the far-wrist activities. From our experimental results from all 20 participants, we find that a short time period $\mathcal{W} = 10\,\text{s}$ is sufficient to cover the duration of typical arm movements, and the threshold $\theta_{\text{ma}} = 30\%$ is general enough to provide high accuracy of categorizing the arm movements for all participants. In our evaluation, we apply this general threshold for categorizing the movements.

8.4.3 Motion Artifacts Removal for Near-wrist Activities

When the system determines that the PPG segments are affected by the near-wrist activities, it implies that the PPG measurements are significantly distorted by the MA during the time in the sliding window, which we consider unrecoverable. In this case, we remove all the PPG segments affected by MA and only perform user authentication using the rest of the PPG segments in the sliding window. However, we find that the PPG segments affected by MA may not be continuous, and the interval between two affected segments may be too short (e.g., $1 \sim 2\,\text{s}$ including $1 \sim 3$ PPG segments) for extracting a complete pulse waveform that can be used to perform user authentication. Hence, we remove all the PPG segments in between the first and last segments affected by MA and keep the unaffected PPG segments for user authentication.

An example of our MA removal for the near-wrist activity is shown in Fig. 8.7a. Based on the MA detection results (i.e., 7 out of all the 12 PPG segments are determined as MA), we can determine the PPG measurements in the sliding window contains the near-wrist activity. Thus, our system removes the PPG segments affected by MA (i.e., from PPG segment index 3 $\sim$ 10) between the first and last detected MA in this sliding window.

As shown in Fig. 8.7b, our MA removal method can successfully remove the PPG measurements that are impacted by the near-wrist activities with respect to the ground truth. In addition, it should be noted that our CA system could still authenticate the user when the hand is stable before/after the near-wrist activities, and removing the MA caused by the near-wrist activities does not influence the user experience since user authentication can be done before the near-wrist activities.

8.4.4 Motion Artifacts Mitigation for Far-wrist Activities

When the system determines that the PPG segments are affected by the far-wrist activities, we notice that the interference of MA is usually small and recoverable. Therefore, we employ a special moving average filter (SMAF) to mitigate those MA and retain them for continuous authentication. The basic idea is to average each recognized MA with several pure pulse segments (i.e., the typical PPG segments without MA) of the current testing user. Then the MA is able to be mitigated from the averaged results. Specifically, we first align the pure pulse PPG segments using the systolic peaks in order to maintain the locations of the critical fiducial points. Since the number of the samples in each pulse segment is not equal, we then interpolate those PPG segments to make them have the same length. After the interpolation, we will apply the SMAF on the pure pulse segments and MA using the following equation:

$$\mathbf{S} = \frac{\sum_{h=1}^{N} \overrightarrow{P_h} + \overrightarrow{M}}{N+1}, \tag{8.2}$$

where the $\overrightarrow{P_h}$ represents the pure pulse segments, $\overrightarrow{M}$ is MA that requires the mitigation, and totally N pure pulse segments and 1 MA are averaged with the mitigated result as $\mathbf{S}$. In particular, we use 4 pure pulse segments for the proposed SMAF. After the SMAF, we use the smooth function to ensure the continuity of the filtered signal. Figure 8.8 illustrates the effectiveness of our MA mitigation for a far-wrist activity, which is raising forearm to check the time. From Fig. 8.8a, we can see that a small proportion of PPG measurements (i.e., the measurements highlighted in red) are affected by the far-wrist activities and detected by our MA detection method. Figure 8.8b presents the results after applying the SMFA filter on the PPG measurements, which can mitigate the impact and reconstruct the pulse waveform.

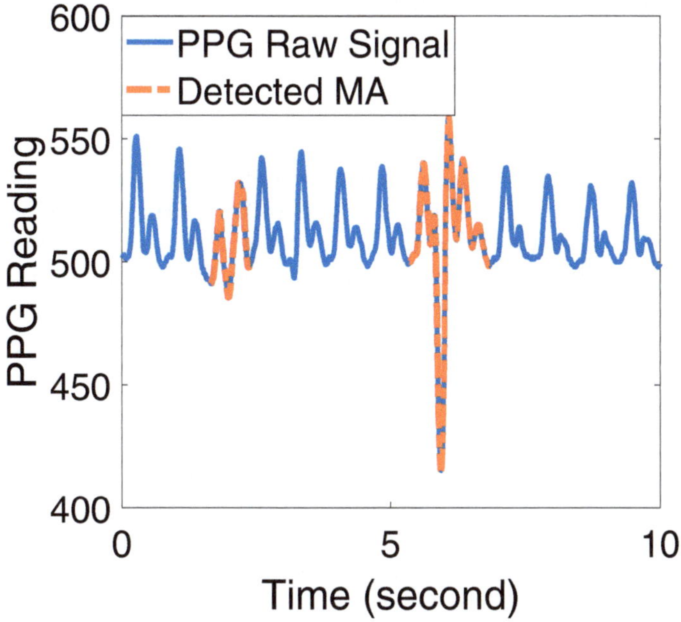

(a)

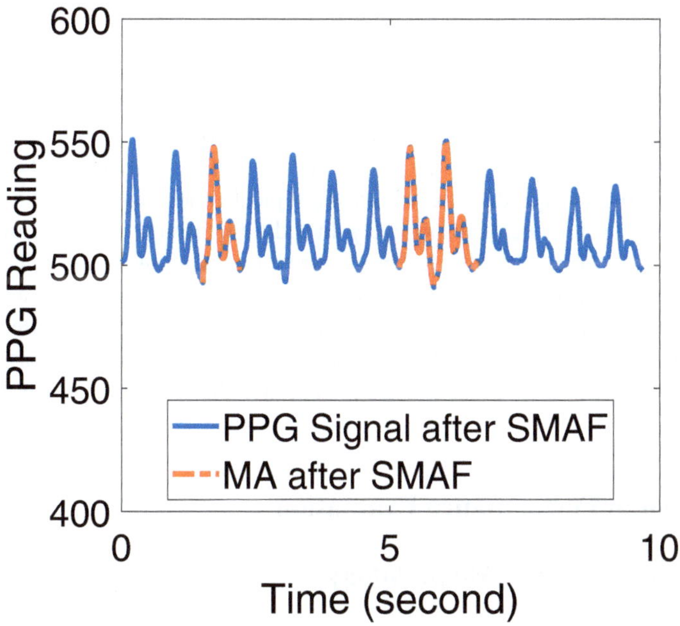

(b)

Fig. 8.8 Example of the MA mitigation using SMAF. (**a**) Raw PPG measurements and detected MA. (**b**) PPG measurements after SMAF filtering

8.5 System Implementation

8.5.1 Data Preprocessing

The PPG measurements from the low-cost PPG sensor in wrist-worn wearable devices inevitably contain baseline drift and high-frequency interference. Since the frequency of the pulsatile component in PPG is $0.5 - 4$ Hz, and the frequency of MA is 0.1 Hz and above, our system firstly applies a band-pass filter to reduce the effect of the baseline drift and high-frequency noise. In particular, we implement a Butterworth bandpass filter with the passband $0.5 - 6$ Hz and the order as 2 to only retain the pulsatile components together with the MA components having a similar spectrum.

8.5.2 Pulse Segmentation

Our system determines the starting and ending points of all the PPG segments in the sliding window. Figure 8.2 shows that the starting and ending points of a typical complete cardiac cycle correspond to the two valley points before the systolic and after diastolic points, respectively. Ideally, we can find all the valley points in the sliding window and extract the data between every two valley points as the PPG segments. However, we find that the dicrotic notch could have the lowest amplitude (i.e., "fake" valley) in the cardiac cycle. Particularly, we tackle this issue based on the fact that the time distances from the systolic peak to the starting and ending points are in the range of $T_s = 0.15\sim 0.26$ s and $T_e = 0.44 \sim 0.74$ s, respectively [5]. Therefore, the accurate PPG segment can be extracted by selecting the valleys that are within the typical time ranges T_s and T_e before and after each systolic peak, respectively. In addition, through our experiments with 20 participants, we empirically determine the sliding window as 2 s larger than one typical pulse waveform (e.g., $0.6 \sim 1$ s) to ensure the effectiveness and accuracy of the PPG segmentation. We also note that our segmentation method is effective with MA because the system finds PPG segments in the sliding window based on the peaks and valleys that fulfill the criteria even though the waveform may be distorted.

8.6 System Performance Evaluation

8.6.1 Experimental Methodology

Wearable Prototype We notice that existing commodity wearable devices can only provide the computed heart rate instead of direct access to raw PPG readings. Therefore, we design a wrist-worn PPG sensing prototype as shown in Fig. 8.9,

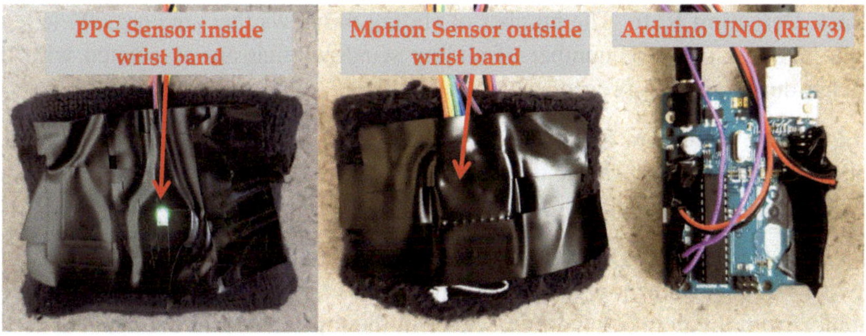

Fig. 8.9 Prototype: wrist-worn PPG sensing platform

which refers to the layout of PPG and motion sensors in commodity wrist-worn wearable device (e.g., Apple Watch). Specifically, the prototype consists of one commodity green LED PPG sensor attached to the inner side of the wristband and a motion sensor (i.e., accelerometer) attached to the outside of the wristband. These sensors are connected to an Arduino UNO (REV3) board for the sensor measurements acquisition, which is under a 300 Hz sampling rate. The PPG measurements are transferred to a laptop (i.e., Dell Latitude E6430) to perform user authentication.

Data Collection We recruit 20 healthy participants whose ages are between 20 to 40 to collect PPG measurements using our wearable prototype. Two different scenarios are adopted to evaluate our system for various practical application scenarios: In the *static scenario*, 20 participants are asked to sit quietly for 10 min. While in the *moving scenario*, we ask 5 participants to perform the *far-wrist activities* (i.e., moving the forearms) and the *near-wrist activities* (i.e., grabbing up a cup and drinking water) repeatedly for 2 mins and sit still for 3 mins. In total, we collect around 15,000 PPG pulse segments from these participants' wrists in the static-scenario and 4200 pulse segments in the moving-scenario, respectively. In addition, we also test our system on the IEEE TBME Benchmark dataset [17], which has 8-min PPG data collected from the fingertips of 42 people with a sampling rate of 300 Hz.

8.6.2 Evaluation Metrics

Our system periodically authenticate the user based on the PPG segments in a sliding window and labels the sliding window as the user or attacker, respectively. We define our evaluation metrics as follows:

CA Accuracy The number of sliding windows that are correctly labeled as the user over the total number of sliding windows that are examined during the CA process.

Attack Detection Rate The number of sliding windows that are correctly labeled as the attacker over the number of sliding windows that are associated with the attacker during the CA process.

Attack False Detection Rate The number of sliding windows that are incorrectly identified as the attacker over the number of sliding windows that are associated with the user during the CA process.

Receiver Operating Characteristic (ROC) Curve It reflects the trade-off between Attack Detection Rate and Attack False Detection Rate. The smallest distance from the point on the ROC curve to the top-left corner corresponds to the optimum model.

In our evaluation, 20 rounds of Monte Carlo cross-validation are employed for the 10-min of the collected user data, among which 5-min for training and the rest of the data for authentication.

8.6.3 Continuous Authentication Performance

We first evaluate the general performance of the system by examining the CA accuracy in the static scenario. In particular, we consider each participant acts as a legitimate user once while remaining participants act as attackers. Figure 8.10a shows that each user achieves comparable high CA accuracy with an average of 90.73% CA accuracy, which indicates that our system can successfully authenticate users with high accuracy using the wrist-worn wearable devices. In addition, Fig. 8.10b shows that our system can achieve even better performance on the PPG data from the fingertip [17] with 39 out of 42 people having the CA accuracy above 96%. This is because the PPG measurements from fingertips are stronger and more stable than those from wrists. These results not only demonstrate the promising practical usability of our proposed user authentication system on common wrist-worn wearable devices but also indicate that it has promising usage in clinical environments such as telemedicine and smart-health applications.

Moreover, to study the performance of our system when defending against the random attack, Fig. 8.11 shows that the ROC curve gets closer to the point (0, 1) when the number of the PPG segments in a sliding window becomes larger. Particularly, our attack detection rate reaches to over 88% with the attack false detection rate of around 3.9% when the length of the sliding window is 4. And our system can achieve over 90% attack detection rate and less than 4.2% attack false detection rate with six or more PPG segments in a sliding window. Those results show that our CA system is robust against the random attacks.

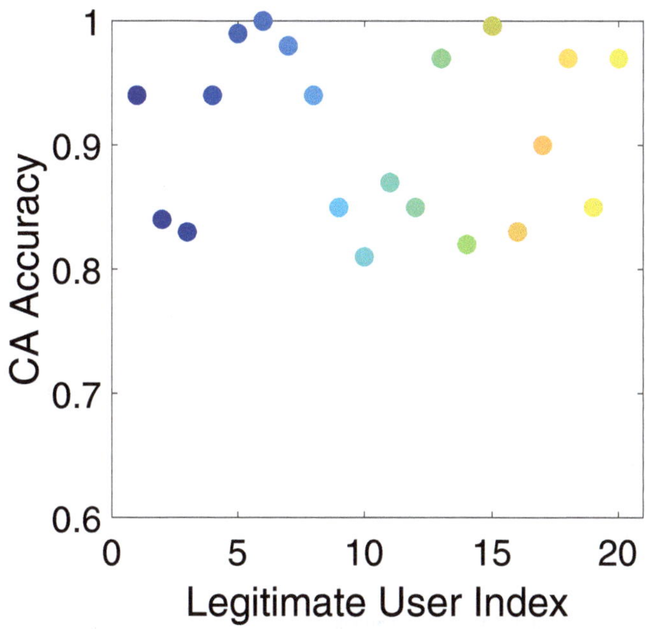

(a)

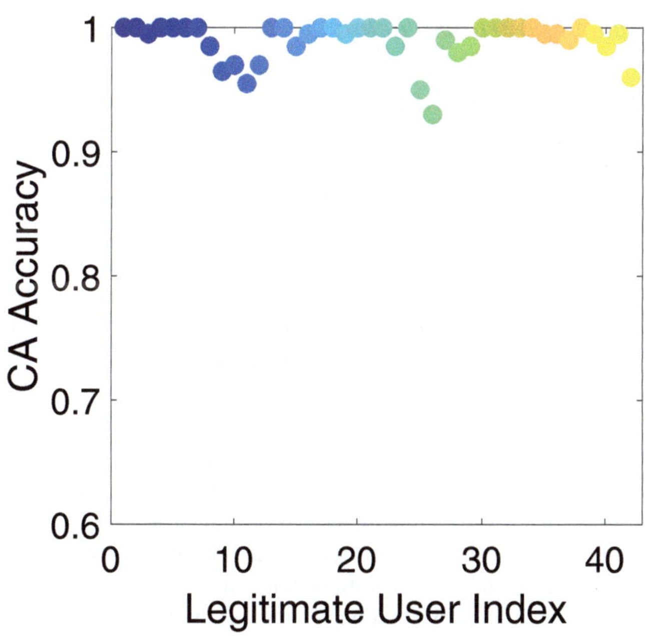

(b)

Fig. 8.10 CA accuracy of our system using the PPG measurements from the wrist areas and the fingertips. (**a**) PPG from the wrist area. (**b**) PPG from the fingertip

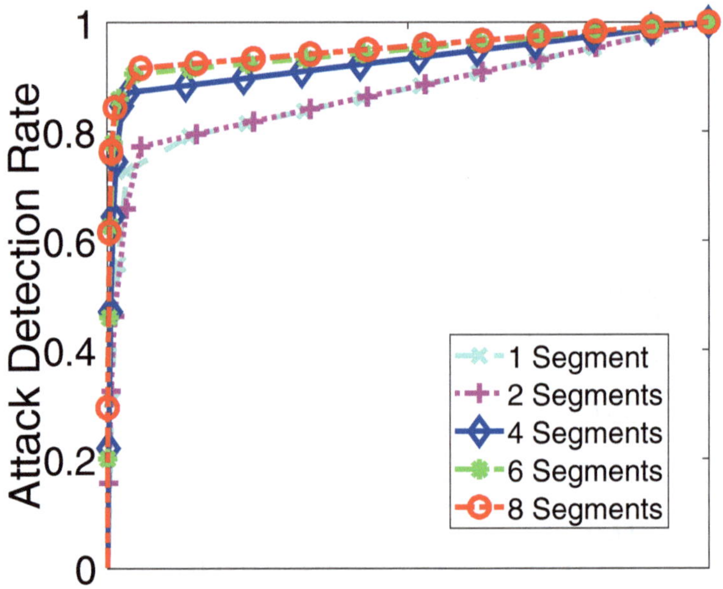

Fig. 8.11 ROC curves under the random attack

8.6.4 *Impact of Various Factors*

Impact of the Sliding Window Length The length of the sliding window corresponds to the number of continuous PPG segments to perform the majority vote for user authentication. Particularly, we test the different lengths of the sliding window with 1, 2, 4, 6, 8 continuous PPG segments (i.e., about 0.7, 1.4, 3, 4.4, and 6 s). Figure 8.12 shows the CA accuracy increases as the increment of the sliding window length and becomes stable at about 90% with four or more PPG segments. Therefore, we adopt the sliding window with 4 continuous PPG segments in our system, which not only provides the high CA accuracy but also has the short response time for the authentication (i.e., around 3 s).

Impact of Training Data Size Since the training data size influences the ease of use in terms of the time for data collection, so we particularly test 1, 2, 3, 4, 5, and 6 min static PPG signals of each user for training respectively, and use the rest data for testing. Figure 8.13a shows that an average CA accuracy of 77.75% is achieved only using 1 min data of each user for training. Moreover, the average CA accuracy can increase to 90.65% and becomes stable when using 5 min or more training data of each user. Those results prove that our system is suitable for practical use since it can achieve very high CA accuracy with the only limited size of training data (e.g., 5-min per user).

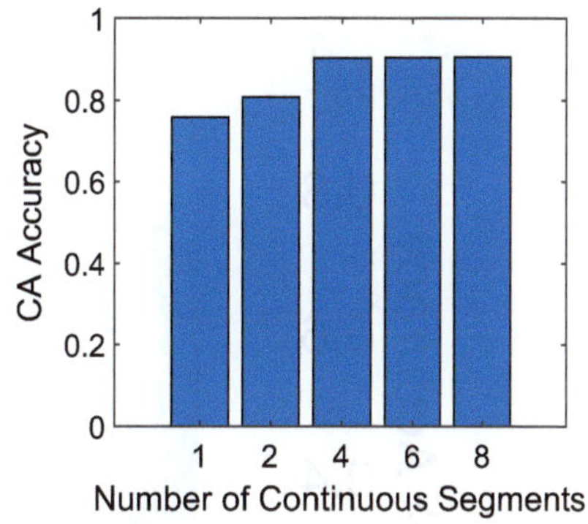

Fig. 8.12 Performance with different lengths of the sliding window

Impact of Machine Learning Methods We study the performance of our system with different underlying machine learning models. Specifically, we adopt the support vector machine (SVM) and neural network (NN) using the LIBSVM library [9] and the multi-layer perceptron in Scikit-learn [25], respectively. Figure 8.13b shows that GBT has the best CA accuracy of 90% compared with SVM (scaling the data) and NN whose CA accuracy is 75 and 80% respectively. This result indicates that GBT easily tuned with flexible optimization options is more suitable for our CA system than the machine learning methods which either are difficult to determine the appropriate kernel (e.g., SVM) or require a large amount of training data and expertise to tune the model (e.g., NN).

Impact of Sampling Rate The sampling rate affects the power consumption and computational cost in the wearable devices. In particular, we find that the CA accuracy is as high as 88% at the lowest sampling rate (i.e., 25 Hz) and increases slightly with the increased sampling rate and becomes stable with 90.7% CA accuracy since 100 Hz. Those findings imply that our CA system is not only compatible with the commodity wrist-worn wearable devices (e.g., Samsung Simband [32] adopts 128 Hz PPG sampling rate) but also supports the hardware with even lower PPG sampling rate.

Performance with Motion Artifacts Removal and Mitigation We next study the performance of our MA removal method on near-wrist activities and MA mitigation method on far-wrist activities among 5 participants, respectively. As shown in Fig. 8.14, while performing far-wrist activities such as moving forearm, our system could still achieve 72.2% CA accuracy even without applying the MA mitigation method and the CA accuracy increases to 89.2% after MA mitigation. Furthermore, we can see that our system has the CA accuracy as 36.6% before MA removal and achieve 75.2% after MA removal for the near-wrist activities such as grabbing up a cup to mimic drinking water gesture. Those results show that the far-wrist activities have a relatively slight impact on our CA system, whereas the near-wrist activities have more impacts due to the involvement of the tendon and muscle in

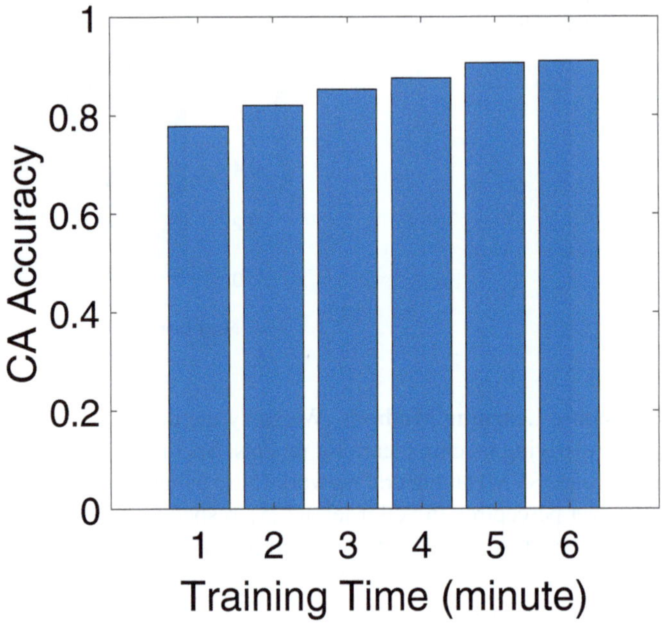

(a)

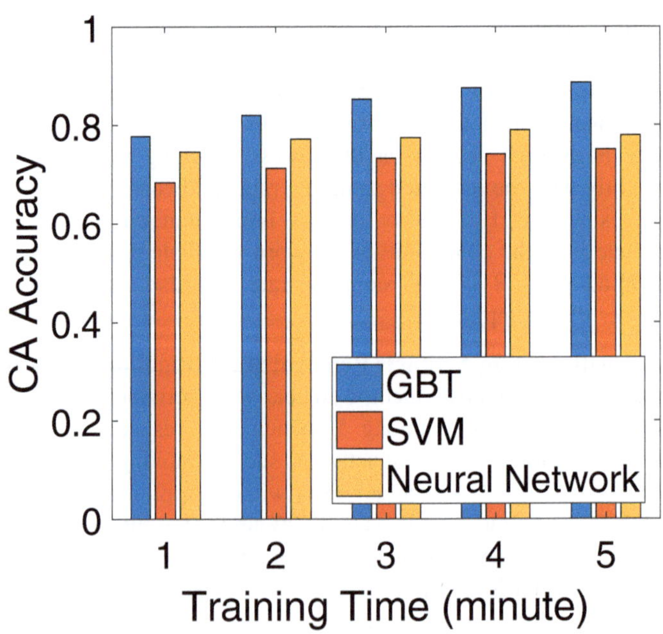

(b)

Fig. 8.13 The impacts of the training size and the machine learning method. (**a**) Performance with different sizes of the training data. (**b**) Performance with different machine learning methods

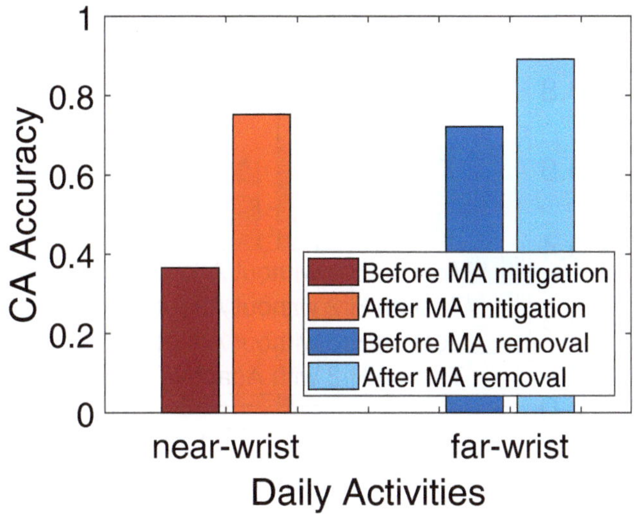

Fig. 8.14 Performance of MA removal

the wrist area. Overall, our system has a decent performance after applying the MA removal method on the near-wrist activities and MA mitigation method on the far-wrist activities, which implies that it's practical for daily life usage.

8.6.5 Effectiveness of Adaptive Training

We evaluate our adaptive training using the data collected by one user across three different hours in a day. Specifically, we collect 1 hour PPG data starting at 11 AM, 1 PM, and 4 PM, respectively. In Fig. 8.15, $Tr1$ represents the training set is only from the first hour and Tr_2 represents the mixed training set includes the data from both the first hour and 2 mins' data from the third hour. We can see that our system trained by $Tr1$ can achieve 91% CA accuracy during the first hour, and decreases 5% during the second hour and 7% during the third hour, respectively. These results demonstrate that the user cardiac system indeed has some fluctuations during a long-time period that slightly impact the CA performance. Moreover, after the adaptive retraining with Tr_2, the CA accuracy will increase back to 90% during the third hour. Those results prove that our system is suitable for long-time user authentication with few times of adaptively retraining which requires a very small amount of the new data. (e.g., routinely retrain every 3 h with only 2 min new data).

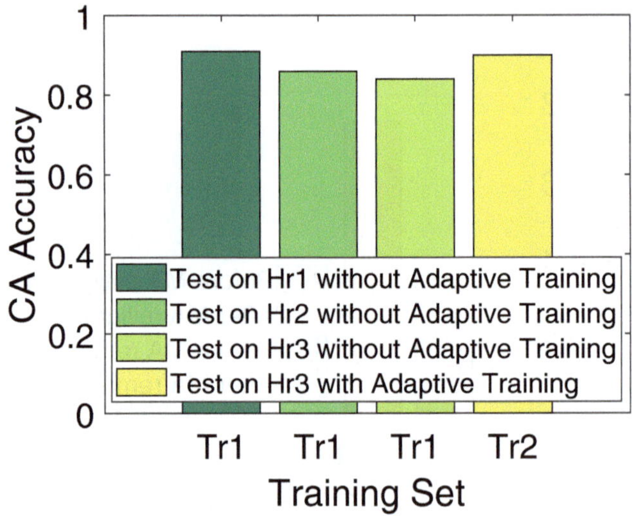

Fig. 8.15 Performance comparison with different testing data with and without adaptive training

8.7 Summary

As an important means for human-computer interactions, gesture recognition has attracted significant research efforts in recent years. This chapter serves as the first step towards a comprehensive understanding of the PPG-based gesture recognition. We made a novel proposition to recognize the fine-grained finger-level gestures such as sign language using low-cost PPG sensors in wearables. In particular, we develop a fine-grained data segmentation method that can successfully separate the unique gesture-related patterns from the PPG measurements that are continuously interfered by pulses. Additionally, we study the unique PPG features resulted from finger-level gestures in different signal domains and devise a system that can effectively recognize finger-level gestures by only using PPG measurements. Our experiments with over 3600 gestures collected from 10 demonstrate that our system can differentiate nine elementary finger-level gestures from American Sign Language with an average recognition accuracy over 88%. We are aware of the intensity of reflected light captured by PPG sensors are sensitive to different skin colors (e.g., light colored skin reflects more light) and locations (e.g., outer side of the wrist has weaker signals); the PPG signals could be significantly impacted by strenuous exercises. We would like to present our findings and seek solutions (e.g., including motion sensors) for these potential impact factors in our future work.

References

1. Al Abdulwahid, A., Clarke, N., Stengel, I., Furnell, S., Reich, C.: A survey of continuous and transparent multibiometric authentication systems. In: European Conference on Cyber Warfare and Security, pp. 1–10 (2015)
2. Aviv, A.J., Gibson, K.L., Mossop, E., Blaze, M., Smith, J.M.: Smudge attacks on smartphone touch screens. Woot **10**, 1–7 (2010)
3. Becker, C., Rigamonti, R., Lepetit, V., Fua, P.: Supervised feature learning for curvilinear structure segmentation. In: International Conference on Medical Image Computing and Computer-Assisted Intervention, pp. 526–533. Springer (2013)
4. Bhargav-Spantzel, A., Squicciarini, A.C., Modi, S., Young, M., Bertino, E., Elliott, S.J.: Privacy preserving multi-factor authentication with biometrics. J. Comput. Secur. **15**(5), 529–560 (2007)
5. Bombardini, T., Gemignani, V., Bianchini, E., Venneri, L., Petersen, C., Pasanisi, E., Pratali, L., Alonso-Rodriguez, D., Pianelli, M., Faita, F., et al.: Diastolic time–frequency relation in the stress echo lab: filling timing and flow at different heart rates. Cardiovasc. Ultrasound **6**(1), 15 (2008)
6. Bonissi, A., Labati, R.D., Perico, L., Sassi, R., Scotti, F., Sparagino, L.: A preliminary study on continuous authentication methods for photoplethysmographic biometrics. In: 2013 IEEE Workshop on Biometric Measurements and Systems for Security and Medical Applications (BIOMS), pp. 28–33. IEEE (2013)
7. Camara, C., Peris-Lopez, P., Gonzalez-Manzano, L., Tapiador, J.: Real-time electrocardiogram streams for continuous authentication. Appl. Soft Comput. **68**, 784–794 (2018)
8. Casale, P., Pujol, O., Radeva, P.: Personalization and user verification in wearable systems using biometric walking patterns. Pers. Ubiquitous Comput. **16**(5), 563–580 (2012)
9. Chang, C.C., Lin, C.J.: LIBSVM: a library for support vector machines. ACM Trans. Intell. Syst. Technol. **2**, 27:1–27:27 (2011). Software available at http://www.csie.ntu.edu.tw/~cjlin/libsvm
10. Elgendi, M.: On the analysis of fingertip photoplethysmogram signals. Curr. Cardiol. Rev. **8**(1), 14–25 (2012)
11. Galar, M., Fernández, A., Barrenechea, E., Bustince, H., Herrera, F.: An overview of ensemble methods for binary classifiers in multi-class problems: Experimental study on one-vs-one and one-vs-all schemes. Pattern Recognit. **44**(8), 1761–1776 (2011)
12. Guennoun, M., Abbad, N., Talom, J., Rahman, S.M.M., El-Khatib, K.: Continuous authentication by electrocardiogram data. In: Proceedings of the 2009 IEEE Toronto International Conference Science and Technology for Humanity (IEEE TIC-STH), pp. 40–42 (2009)
13. Hastie, T., Tibshirani, R., Friedman, J.: The Elements of Statistical Learning. Springer, New York (2009)
14. Kang, S.J., Lee, S.Y., Cho, H.I., Park, H.: Ecg authentication system design based on signal analysis in mobile and wearable devices. IEEE Signal Process. Lett. **23**(6), 805–808 (2016)
15. Karimian, N., Guo, Z., Tehranipoor, M., Forte, D.: Human recognition from photoplethysmography (ppg) based on non-fiducial features. In: Proceedings of the 2017 IEEE International Conference on Acoustics, Speech and Signal Processing (IEEE ICASSP), pp. 4636–4640 (2017)
16. Karimian, N., Tehranipoor, M., Forte, D.: Non-fiducial ppg-based authentication for healthcare application. In: Proceedings of the 2017 IEEE EMBS International Conference on Biomedical & Health Informatics (BHI) (IEEE EMBS), pp. 429–432 (2017)
17. Karlen, W., Raman, S., Ansermino, J.M., Dumont, G.A.: Multiparameter respiratory rate estimation from the photoplethysmogram. IEEE Trans. Biomed. Eng. **60**(7), 1946–1953 (2013)
18. Kavsaoğlu, A.R., Polat, K., Bozkurt, M.R.: A novel feature ranking algorithm for biometric recognition with ppg signals. Comput. Biol. Med. **49**, 1–14 (2014)

19. Lashkari, A.H., Farmand, S., Zakaria, D., Bin, O., Saleh, D., et al.: Shoulder surfing attack in graphical password authentication. Preprint (2009). arXiv:0912.0951
20. Lin, F., Song, C., Zhuang, Y., Xu, W., Li, C., Ren, K.: Cardiac scan: a non-contact and continuous heart-based user authentication system. In: Proceedings of the 23rd Annual International Conference on Mobile Computing and Networking (ACM MobiCom), pp. 315–328 (2017)
21. Mare, S., Markham, A.M., Cornelius, C., Peterson, R., Kotz, D.: Zebra: zero-effort bilateral recurring authentication. In: 2014 IEEE Symposium on Security and Privacy (SP), pp. 705–720. IEEE (2014)
22. Mondol, M.A.S., Emi, I.A., Preum, S.M., Stankovic, J.A.: User authentication using wrist mounted inertial sensors. In: Proceedings of the 16th ACM/IEEE International Conference on Information Processing in Sensor Networks, pp. 309–310 (2017)
23. Niu, X., Han, H., Shan, S., Chen, X.: Continuous heart rate measurement from face: a robust rppg approach with distribution learning. In: 2017 IEEE International Joint Conference on Biometrics (IJCB), pp. 642–650. IEEE (2017)
24. Ometov, A., Bezzateev, S., Mäkitalo, N., Andreev, S., Mikkonen, T., Koucheryavy, Y.: Multi-factor authentication: a survey. Cryptography **2**(1), 1 (2018)
25. Pedregosa, F., Varoquaux, G., Gramfort, A., Michel, V., Thirion, B., Grisel, O., Blondel, M., Prettenhofer, P., Weiss, R., Dubourg, V., Vanderplas, J., Passos, A., Cournapeau, D., Brucher, M., Perrot, M., Duchesnay, E.: Scikit-learn: Machine learning in Python. J. Mach. Learn. Res. **12**, 2825–2830 (2011)
26. Pinto, J.R., Cardoso, J.S., Lourenço, A., Carreiras, C.: Towards a continuous biometric system based on ecg signals acquired on the steering wheel. Sensors **17**(10), 2228 (2017)
27. Pu, L., Chacon, P.J., Wu, H.C., Choi, J.W.: Novel tailoring algorithm for abrupt motion artifact removal in photoplethysmogram signals. Biomed. Eng. Lett. **7**(4), 299–304 (2017)
28. Rahman, A., Lubecke, V., Boric-Lubecke, O., Prins, J., Sakamoto, T.: Doppler radar techniques for accurate respiration charac-terization and subject identification. IEEE J. Emerg. Sel. Top. Circuits Syst. **8**, 350–359 (2018)
29. Ren, Y., Chen, Y., Chuah, M.C., Yang, J.: User verification leveraging gait recognition for smartphone enabled mobile healthcare systems. IEEE Trans. Mobile Comput. **14**(9), 1961–1974 (2015)
30. Sarkar, A., Abbott, A.L., Doerzaph, Z.: Biometric authentication using photoplethysmography signals. In: 2016 IEEE 8th International Conference on Biometrics Theory, Applications and Systems (BTAS), pp. 1–7. IEEE (2016)
31. Shepherd, J.T., Vanhoutte, P.M.: The Human Cardiovascular System: Facts and Concepts. Raven Press, New York (1979)
32. Simband: Why is 128 hz used as a sampling frequency for the ppg signals? (2017). http://www.simband.io/documentation/faq.html
33. Traore, I., Woungang, I., Obaidat, M.S., Nakkabi, Y., Lai, I.: Combining mouse and keystroke dynamics biometrics for risk-based authentication in web environments. In: Proceedings of the Fourth International Conference on Digital Home Digital Home (IEEE ICDH), pp. 138–145 (2012)

Chapter 9
Conclusion and Future Directions

In this chapter, we summarize the main research results of using mobile technologies for smart healthcare presented in this book and highlight the potential future research directions.

9.1 Conclusion

In summary, this book provides a comprehensive exploration of the inventive applications of mobile technologies in transforming the healthcare industry. Among numerous technologies, WiFi has emerged as one of today's most prevalent technologies, enabling the smart healthcare system in addition to its original usage for communication purposes. We started with an overview of a system engineered to recognize location-based activities by leveraging the widespread presence of WiFi infrastructure. We then examined the design of a personalized fitness assistant system, applicable in both residential and professional environments, leveraging the existing WiFi infrastructure. We also explored the utilization of millimeter wave (mmWave) technology, the most advanced wireless technology, showcasing our work on the design and implementation of a fitness assistant system using a single off-the-shelf mmWave device. Recognizing the vital role of nutrition in health, we developed a non-intrusive eating habit monitoring system. This system aims to consistently monitor eating behaviors, regardless of the surroundings.

In addition to wireless solutions, we extended the original usage of wearables to have a deeper usage in the mobile health area. Along this line, we showed that personalized fitness assistant systems can be designed and developed using smartphones or smartwatches. We demonstrated the concept of a virtual fitness assistant system using wearables designed to promote effective workouts while minimizing the risk of injuries. This system provides a dynamic view of a user's short-term and long-term exercise activities, drawing data from sensors in wearable

X. Guo et al., *Mobile Technologies for Smart Healthcare System Design*, Wireless Networks, https://doi.org/10.1007/978-3-031-57345-3_9

mobile devices. Lastly, we discussed advanced healthcare applications facilitated by photoplethysmography (PPG) sensors found commonly on mobile devices. We illustrated how to utilize built-in PPG sensors on wrist-worn wearable devices for intricate finger-level gesture recognition, sign language interpretation, and continuous user authentication. In short, this book has covered a wide array of technological advancements and their impact on smart healthcare, signifying the promising potential at the crossroads of technology and health.

9.2 Future Directions

A promising direction for future research is to study the security vulnerabilities of deep learning (DL) techniques used in mobile health technologies. As DL becomes integral to mobile healthcare systems, these systems may become vulnerable to sophisticated cyber threats in the form of adversarial attacks. Therefore, developing robust DL models that can detect, withstand, and recover from adversarial attacks is critical for securing mobile health data and systems. Specific areas of research could include designing novel algorithms to identify and mitigate adversarial attacks against DL models, as well as exploring training strategies and architectures that enhance the security and resilience of DL models used in healthcare applications.

Another promising area of research is developing mobile health technologies that can adapt to dynamic environmental changes. Mobile healthcare systems usually operate under diverse and often unpredictable conditions, making adaptability critical for maintaining performance and reliability. This situation presents an opportunity to explore self-adjusting mobile health technologies that can optimally respond to real-time environmental fluctuations. Potential research directions include leveraging machine learning and artificial intelligence to create intelligent systems that automatically adjust their operation based on environmental changes. Such research could involve training models to detect meaningful shifts in parameters like available network bandwidth, computing resources, ambient lighting, or noise levels and then accordingly implement compensatory changes to sensing, processing, or interface configurations.

The third emerging research direction in smart health technologies focuses on creating integrated systems for comprehensive health monitoring and personalized medicine. These systems will enable advanced healthcare applications that exploit long-term monitoring to improve disease prevention and treatment, including telemedicine, customized treatments, and remote healthcare services. By synergizing various mobile sensing modalities, researchers can develop interconnected systems that monitor a wide array of health metrics (e.g., vital signs, physical activity, and sleep patterns), offering a holistic view of an individual's health. Advanced signal processing techniques and data analytic algorithms could be developed to process and analyze such data, enabling early detection of health risks, personalized health interventions, and optimized treatment plans. The essential goal of this direction is to move beyond reactive healthcare towards a more proactive, preventive, and personalized approach. The integrated smart health systems would not only empower individuals to manage their health more effectively but also provide healthcare professionals with deeper insights for better patient care. Research in this area holds the promise of transforming healthcare delivery by making it more responsive, efficient, and tailored to individual needs.

MIX
Papier aus verantwortungsvollen Quellen
Paper from responsible sources
FSC® C105338

If you have any concerns about our products,
you can contact us on
ProductSafety@springernature.com

In case Publisher is established outside the EU,
the EU authorized representative is:
Springer Nature Customer Service Center GmbH
Europaplatz 3, 69115 Heidelberg, Germany

Printed by Libri Plureos GmbH
in Hamburg, Germany